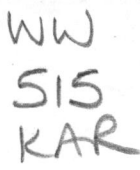

A Systematic
Approach
to Strabismus

Second Edition

A Systematic Approach to Strabismus

Second Edition

Virginia C. Karlsson, CO, COMT
Certified Orthoptist
Mayo Clinic
Rochester, Minnesota

Series Editors:

Janice K. Ledford • Ken Daniels • Robert Campbell

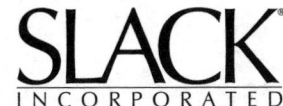

SLACK ®
INCORPORATED
Delivering the best in health care information and education worldwide

www.slackbooks.com

ISBN: 978-1-55642-794-7

The procedures and practices described in this book should be implemented in a manner consistent with the professional standards set for the circumstances that apply in each specific situation. Every effort has been made to confirm the accuracy of the information presented and to correctly relate generally accepted practices. The authors, editor, and publisher cannot accept responsibility for errors or exclusions or for the outcome of the material presented herein. There is no expressed or implied warranty of this book or information imparted by it. Care has been taken to ensure that drug selection and dosages are in accordance with currently accepted/recommended practice. Due to continuing research, changes in government policy and regulations, and various effects of drug reactions and interactions, it is recommended that the reader carefully review all materials and literature provided for each drug, especially those that are new or not frequently used. Any review or mention of specific companies or products is not intended as an endorsement by the author or publisher.

SLACK Incorporated uses a review process to evaluate submitted material. Prior to publication, educators or clinicians provide important feedback on the content that we publish. We welcome feedback on this work.

Published by: SLACK Incorporated
                    6900 Grove Road
                    Thorofare, NJ 08086 USA
                    Telephone: 856-848-1000
                    Fax: 856-848-6091
                    www.slackbooks.com

Contact SLACK Incorporated for more information about other books in this field or about the availability of our books from distributors outside the United States.

Library of Congress Cataloging-in-Publication Data

Karlsson, Virginia.
  A systematic approach to strabismus / Virginia Karlsson. -- 2nd ed.
      p. ; cm.
  Includes bibliographical references and index.
  ISBN-13: 978-1-55642-794-7 (alk. paper)
  ISBN-10: 1-55642-794-8 (alk. paper)
  1. Strabismus. 2. Eye--Examination. 3. Ophthalmic assistants. I. Title.
  [DNLM: 1. Strabismus. 2. Strabismus--diagnosis. WW 415 K18s 2008]
  RE771.H36 2008
  617.7'62--dc22
                                2008029541

Printed in the United States of America.

Last digit is print number: 10 9 8 7 6 5 4 3 2 1

Dedication

In memory of
Steven William Salevouris

1956 – 2006

Orthoptist, technologist, student, true gentleman, and friend.

Contents

Acknowledgments

Another 10 or so years have gone by since *A Systematic Approach to Strabismus* was first written for SLACK in response to their success with the original 12-volume series for ophthalmic personnel. Now, we have this second edition: my third book, but probably not the last.

Again, I've learned a lot in the past 10 years and am grateful to the pediatric ophthalmologists at the Mayo Clinic with whom I've had the pleasure to work. They have encouraged me to have the best of both worlds: seeing real patients within a team approach and teaching and academics. Drs. Jonathan Holmes, Michael Brodsky, Brian Mohney, and George Hohberger all have shared a common joy in the care of our patients and a wonderful variety in styles of doing so!

I blinked, and it happened: my children have grown up considerably. Thank you Dory for proving that the impossible can happen. Thank you Lars for taking on an impossible role. Thank you Carlson for fitting in impossible places. Thank you Greta for knowing that everything is possible, and thank you Colby for reminding me daily that today might just possibly be the best.

About the Author

Virginia Carlson's orthoptic career began at the age of 2 when she climbed over into the front seat of her parents' 1956 Chevy Bel Air and gave her mother a corneal abrasion with her fingernail. Unfortunately, this abrasion was to her mother's NON-amblyopic eye and required 3 days of pressure patching to heal. From that point onward, however, her mother always claimed that her amblyopic eye could see just a little bit better after all that albeit unintentional, occlusive therapy that had been overlooked in her childhood.

Virginia Karlsson, now spelling her last name the way her paternal grandfather had before immigrating to the United States, celebrated her 30th year as a certified orthoptist in 2008.

Colby-Sawyer College in New London, New Hampshire, provided her introduction to orthoptics as a career, providing an excellent undergraduate experience. The University of Florida orthoptic training program in Gainesville provided something unique 32 years ago—simultaneous training as a tech and as an orthoptist. After graduating, Carlson now Hansen returned to New England where she took two part-time jobs: one as a tech to support her second part-time job as an orthoptist in western Massachusetts. Two years later, she became the director of the orthoptic training program at Tufts-New England Medical Center in Boston. After the birth of her first child, she filled in (twice each) for other orthoptists out on maternity leave themselves at the University of Massachusetts in Worcester; the Lions Orthoptic Clinic in Springfield, Massachusetts; and the Newington Children's Hospital in Newington, Connecticut.

She returned to work full-time in 1990 when her family moved to Minneapolis; she worked for a large health system and then a private practice. In 2005, Karlsson took the orthoptic position at the Mayo Clinic and has thoroughly enjoyed the extraordinarily challenging patients, the completely ordinary patients, the academic environment, and the peaceful commute from Minneapolis to Rochester, Minnesota.

Five children with varied interests don't leave much time for Mom, but most recently she has remembered how to ski, speak Swedish, play kubb (poorly), and definitely laugh more. "Don't blink!" is the advice she tells new parents about their baby's first year of life. Maybe she shouldn't have blinked so much over the past 30 years of being an orthoptist!

Foreword

Many of us can remember the sense of inadequacy we first felt when we tried to approach a young child to glean any information from his or her eyes. Pediatric ophthalmology and strabismus are "lore unto themselves"; it seems that nothing we learn from examining adults applies to these hypermobile, hyperdistractable bundles of joy. In this book, Ginny Karlsson shares with us many superbly practical tips for "making it happen"; acquiring that information from the child; allowing us to discover, treat, and help; while still having fun. Fun for them and fun for us.

For beginning orthoptists, ophthalmic technicians, and ophthalmology residents, this book is crammed full of helpful pearls and insights based on the many years of Ginny's experience. It has been a joy to work with Ginny taking care of children. May you also find a sense of joy as you embark on the adventure of taking care of children who have eye problems.

Jonathan M. Holmes, MD
Professor and Chair of Ophthalmology
Mayo Clinic
Rochester, Minnesota

Introduction

As an orthoptic student I remember staring at my big, blank exam sheet and wondering what the patient in the exam chair had. Worse was staring at my big filled-in exam sheet and wondering what the patient in the exam chair had. Now I'm looking at a computerized chart note with drop-down boxes of cookie-cutter choices and realize that no matter how much gets filled in, we still have to think about how to put our whole exam together and be able to make sense of the information. Over time (up to the present and beyond), the examination of the patient with strabismus has become clearer to me, and it is that exam that I have tried to put into this book.

Many other texts cover pediatric ophthalmology and strabismus in immense detail. My only intention here is to get the beginner started turning that big, blank exam sheet; computer monitor; or some yet-to-be-invented tool into a skillfully diagnosed patient with a treatment plan that the patient and parents will work with.

Virginia C. Karlsson, CO, COMT
Certified Orthoptist
Mayo Clinic
Rochester, Minnesota

Chapter 1

The Systematic Approach to Strabismus

KEY POINTS

- Visual maturity commonly occurs at 9 years of age.

- Exam pollution is avoided by conducting the exam in a systematic order—history, fusion, alignment, and (finally) vision.

- Practice tests on cooperative adults before attempting to do them on children.

Congratulations! You have bravely entered the world of strabismus and ocular motility. This is the same world that has terrified residents and technicians, brought experienced ophthalmologists to their knees, and placed a smile on the orthoptist's face. This book is designed to get you past the common core of knowledge that you possess and move you boldly into the exam room face-to-face with a 3-year-old child. You know how to test vision and you have read how to measure stereopsis. The technique for doing a prism and cover test really did not sound that difficult. So why the terror when your next chart reads, "3 year old with RET"?

Two Eyes

Strabismus and its related subjects bring the added dimension of a second eye to the eye exam. Although you are always testing two eyes when testing vision, refracting, or testing pressure, each eye is treated as a separate entity. Start thinking of the two eyes as a pair, a combination to be reckoned with as a single unit. Despite familiarity with the basic tests required to complete a motility exam, performing these tests gracefully, accurately, and in an orderly and timely fashion on that 3-year-old child with the right esotropia may be a sticking point in your repertoire of techniques.

Four Hints for the Child's Eye Exam

1. Visual maturity can be your friend or your enemy. Visual maturity refers to that magical age, unique to every individual, at which time the visual system has matured to its full capacity and is no longer malleable. A normal infant's vision develops at a rapid rate after birth, reaching 20/20 adult-like vision by 6 months of age. An infant's control of his or her eye movements should be normal and therefore completely straight by 4 months of age. Both vision and motility, however, continue to change for years to come. While each individual is different, age 9 is commonly cited as the age at which visual maturity frequently occurs. This means that a child's vision may no longer improve after that age if therapy is attempted, and conversely, may no longer be lost if therapy is discontinued at his or her own personal age of visual maturity.

2. Your examination technique must change when examining children or babies. The new set of rules requires speed. The quicker the exam on a child can be accomplished, the better. Measurements are more accurate on a happy, relaxed, and attentive child (and parent). The exam will go considerably smoother on a child who is dazzled by the flurry of activity you perform in front of him or her. When something is happening to the child all of the time and the child is distracted, there is less chance that the child will be uncooperative. In order to do this, you, the examiner, must plan and practice. First, practice the skills you need on cooperative adults; do not waste your time trying to learn on a squirming child. Anticipate the tests you will need to accomplish on this particular individual before you have involved the child in the exam. Plan so as to limit the time the child will actually sit in the chair (my personal preference is always on the parent's lap if under age 5 or 6). To work within this limited amount of time, take your history with the parent/child sitting in regular chairs in the exam room rather than in the exam chair. Once you are completely ready to stop asking the boring questions and get to the fun part of the exam, move the child with parent to the chair, inviting him or her to look at your cool stuff. Do not ever actually say that it is an eye

exam, which puts many children on guard for a frightening experience. If you really want to get the child's attention, speak softly. That will get everyone's attention.

3.   Not every test needs to be done on every patient. Do only those that are necessary. Assuming that your young patient's cooperation will only last a finite period of time, plan on doing that part of the exam that is most necessary while the child is still cooperative. For instance, if a child is destined to be cyclopleged with a postcyclo refraction, do not waste time trying to get a manifest refraction. The tables in Chapter 7 will help you put together an exam strategy.

4.   Try to limit the level of exam pollution. Exam pollution happens when performing one test alters the outcome of a subsequent test. An example of this in general ophthalmology would be to anesthetize the cornea for a pressure check before checking corneal sensitivity. Testing order is critical. A strabismus exam has four key parts: history, vision, alignment measurements, and fusion. But those tests are never done in that order!

Fusion is most easily disturbed by measuring alignment or vision, so fusion is usually measured first. Since the most sensitive fusion test should be done initially, stereopsis is measured first. This would be followed by Worth four-dot testing if desired and then the single cover–uncover test (which does not measure alignment but tests for motor fusion control; for more on this, see Chapter 2).

Ideally, alignment measurement should be done before vision testing, since prolonged patching of the eye for vision testing could alter the everyday ocular alignment and will certainly disrupt fusion. Alignment measurements require the proper fixation target, appropriate measuring test, and your polished technique.

Vision testing on children requires your utmost patience. The ability of the patient must be considered and the appropriate test selected long before the patch goes on the child's eye. An adhesive patch should always be used to prevent cheating and peeking, unintentional or otherwise. Finally, while the patch is still on, a dry retinoscopy or manifest refraction (to be balanced later) should be done, and vision rechecked for improvement, with that correction in place.

You can learn how to do all of this by keeping the guidelines in order and by mastering your skills practicing on cooperative adults.

Chapter 2

The Four-Part Exam

KEY POINTS

- History and observation provide clues to the potential diagnosis.

- The exam is done in a particular order—history first, then fusion, then alignment, and vision last.

- The potential diagnosis determines what additional tests are necessary to complete the exam.

The ocular motility exam generally has four parts, which are performed in the following order: history clues (so you will hopefully know what you are looking for), fusion testing, alignment assessment, and vision. This order of testing is essential to reduce pollution of the test results.

Part 1. History Clues—The Story Begins

Some patients/parents have no idea what is wrong with them/their child. It is our job to attempt to narrow down the differential diagnosis by asking pertinent history questions. The pertinent questions are the ones your doctor would like you to ask. So ask your attending physician just how involved he or she would like your history taking to be. If the doctor does not care about a full-term baby's birth weight, do not waste time asking.

Taking a history allows you to size up both the patient and parent. How accurately does the parent observe the child? Has he or she noticed that 2-year-old Erin tilts her head to the side (which you already noticed in the waiting room)? Or is that a big surprise to the parents? Always ask the child some benign question to determine: A) if the parent will allow his or her child to participate in the exam, and B) if the child will be participating in the exam. All you want is a response, verbal or otherwise, so just ask a yes/no question: "Did you see the goldfish in our tank?" "Did you drive all the way here? ...or did Mommy?" "Do you know these people?" as you smile and gesture to his or her parents.

To assess the child's developmental capabilities, probe further by asking a simple question but one that requires a thoughtful answer. A 2 year old should be able to answer: "How old are you?" or "What's your baby's name?" A 3 to 4 year old should be able to tell you: "Are you plain 3, or 3-and-a-half? How old is your brother?" A 5 to 6 year old should know if he or she is going to school/kindergarten in the fall. A child in first grade and up should respond appropriately to "What grade are you in? What's your teacher's name? Is she nice? Is he smart? Is your teacher fair? What's your favorite thing about second grade?" While all of this sounds like idle chit-chat, you will have gained a wealth of information, particularly about the child's ability to understand your questions; his or her cognition, hearing, and speech/verbal skills; and his or her attitude about school. That attitude in particular is important because a significant number of children are brought in for eye exams by parents who are worried about the child's school performance.

Only ask the questions you need to know, and be extremely specific. Do not ask, "Have you ever had any eye problems?" if you do not care about the minor corneal abrasion the patient had 10 years ago. Do not ask, "Is there any family history of strabismus?" if you want to know "Are there any immediate family members with an eye that turns in, or out, or who had to wear a patch when they were younger?" If you want to know if there are any high myopes in the family, ask specifically if any family members are known to wear strong glasses and at a young age. Then you might try to determine if they were plus or minus.

Use common language. Instead of asking the patient if there is any family history of glaucoma, ask if any family members had high pressure in the eye and had to take eye drops every day. Instead of inquiring if the school was worried about amblyopia, ask if the school found a difference in vision in the two eyes. Instead of asking if the child has any ptosis, ask if one lid is droopy or different from the other.

Ask questions in such a way as to get accurate answers. "What brings you to our office today?" discourages patients from telling about their last eye exam at the mall or the springtime allergies they had 6 months ago. Your job is to determine whether the problem is visual, symptomatic, cosmetic, or a combination of these. Use all of your history-taking skills to probe at any problem: "What makes it better/worse? When did it start? Who notices it?" (Grandparents can be exceedingly accurate regarding grandchildren who they see sporadically with a fresh, albeit scrutinizing eye.)

A child who was able to articulate a visual complaint to his or her parents certainly should be able to intelligently respond to questions put forth by a professional: "When you see the double vision, is it side-to-side like this (demonstrate with your hands) or up and down like this? Is it blurry when you read a book or when you sit at the back of the room and try to read the board or overhead projector? Is it blurry to everyone else in class (because of glare, angle, poor penmanship) or just to you?"

It is often difficult for patients/parents to verbalize medical problems. A parent may be reluctant to blurt out the details of the child's problem(s) in front of the child. A patient is often kept unaware of the diagnosis until it has been confirmed. If you get nowhere when you ask the patient if there are any ongoing health problems, ask what other doctors he or she has seen. The patient may have no idea that the reason he or she is suddenly seeing double, has lost weight, has been sent to see an endocrinologist who did blood work, and now needs a motility/eye exam is because someone thinks that he or she probably has Graves' disease or a thyroid problem. We often encounter patients who deny that they have high blood pressure because they are on medication that controls it. Ask what medications the patient is on, but find out if it is important to know how much medication and what time of day it is taken. You need to know when the patient last took his or her glaucoma drops, but does it really matter when his or her last antihistamine was taken? Knowing which doctors are currently following the patient and what medications the patient is on will help complete the patient's history.

Record the patient's allergies to medication, food, and the environment. Patients often do not realize that an eye drop can actually affect their heart or that an allergy to peanuts could be fatal in a child given the eye drop phospholine iodide.

As far as the parents are concerned, visual history can be divided into two categories: the child needs glasses in order to see properly, or more seriously, the child might have uncorrectable vision and be blind. Amblyopia, which frequently requires occlusion therapy along with glasses, falls halfway between those two categories since although it is only one eye, it results in permanent loss of vision if left untreated. Ask the parents, "How do you think Gus sees?" followed by, "Who wonders if he sees okay?" This will usually get the answers necessary to determine if blindness is a true concern or if the visit is merely due to a failed vision screening in a 4 year old who otherwise appears normal. These questions will usually elicit the parents' real concerns, which range from their genuine fear that their baby is blind to disappointment that their child will be wearing spectacles.

Symptomatic history also has two categories: behavior that is observed (by the parents, teachers, or mother-in-law) and symptoms that the child complains about (cannot see, does not want to go to school, headaches, does not want to go to school, does not want glasses, does not want to go to school, sees double, does not want to go to school). The child's complaints may be real or fictitious. Table 2-1 lists observed behavior and the potential diagnoses. Table 2-2 lists typical childhood complaints.

Cosmetic history immediately implies a surgical correction in the minds of parents and children. An honest response to "How do you think the eyes look?" may be tainted by their fear of surgery. When strabismus is obviously present, ask the child if his or her friends ever say anything about his or her eye alignment. Ask if people who are not the child's friends ever comment on it and if that bothers him or her. Ask the parents who else notices the child's misalignment. The

Table 2-1

Observed Behavior	Potential Diagnosis
Holding objects close/sitting near the TV	Myopia
Intermittent crossing, especially at near	Hyperopia/accommodative esotropia
Tearing/discharge in infant/baby	Nasolacrimal duct obstruction
Tearing/photophobia/large eyes	Congenital glaucoma
Head positioning	Null point for nystagmus
Turning face to one side	Lateral incomitance (Duane syndrome/VI nerve palsy)
Tilting head to one side	IV nerve palsy
Tipping chin up	Avoiding upgaze (Brown syndrome/double elevator palsy/A or V pattern)
Tipping chin down	Avoiding downgaze (A or V pattern)
Headache, diplopia, tires when reading	Convergence insufficiency

Table 2-2

Typical Childhood Complaints	Potential Cause
Blurry: Distance only	Myopia
Near only	Extreme hyperopia or convergence insufficiency
Both	Astigmatism, malingering, or amblyopia
Headache	Any phoria with poor fusional amplitudes
	Convergence insufficiency
Diplopia	Any intermittent deviation with poor control
	Recent appreciation of physiologic diplopia
Strabismus without diplopia	Any tropic or intermittent deviation with suppression
Eyes hurt	Any of the above plus foreign body
Eyes tear while reading	Convergence insufficiency

observational powers of loving parents (and spouses) is remarkably accurate or blind, with some parents noticing a microtropia and others being able to ignore a 40 prism diopter tropia. This is why it is so important to ask the parents who else notices the deviation. The parent who thinks his or her child looks just fine with a 20 prism diopter exotropia (XT) may still consider surgery if other people are constantly noticing it and commenting on it.

Part 2. Fusion—Sensory and Motor

Sensory fusion is the blending of two images, one from each eye, into a single image in the brain. Motor fusion is the effort put forth by the brain and oculomotor system to align the eyes so as to be able to achieve sensory fusion. So motor fusion is not necessary in a patient who has a constant tropia, yet is the hallmark of the patient who has a phoria or intermittent tropia. It is motor fusion that keeps the deviation at best phoric, or at least intermittent.

There are three main methods of measuring sensory fusion: stereo tests, Worth four-dot, and haploscopic devices such as the synoptophore and troposcope.

While some stereo tests, such as the Lang stereo test, do not require polarizing stereo glasses, other tests, such as the Birch Randot or Titmus stereo test, which measures fine grades of stereopsis, do. If you do not get the glasses on the child, you cannot do the test. Every examiner has a style of child-patient coercion. Here are some hints for testing stereopsis that have worked

Table 2-3
Worth Four-Dot (Red Lens Over Right Eye)

Response	Means	Record as
4 lights: 1 red/3 green, 2 red/2 green	Fusion in ortho patient	Fuse
	ARC in tropic patient	
2 red lights only	Left green eye suppressing	OS suppress
3 green lights only	Right red eye suppressing	OD suppress
2 reds, then 3 greens not at same moment	Alternate suppression	Alt suppress
2 reds seen to the right of the 3 greens	Uncrossed (homonymous) diplopia	Unc diplopia
	NRC in ET patient	
	ARC if not ET	
2 reds seen to the left of the 3 greens	Crossed (heteronymous) diplopia	X ed diplopia
	NRC in XT patient	
	ARC if not XT	

ARC = anomalous retinal correspondence; NRC = normal retinal correspondence; ET = esotropia; XT = exotropia

for me. While holding the test booklet and ready to start asking about the animals, I inform the child that "we" will be putting on the very cool glasses (and I have got the glasses on the child by now) so that the child can show Mommy or Daddy just how cool her or she is. (I am rambling in whispers by now, but that keeps the child from thinking about taking off the glasses.) "And now, you can see the animals. Does one of them (without taking a breath) look like it's sticking up at you, like it's sticking up off of the page? (Do not wait for an answer.) Push it down for me, push him back down on the page. (Ignore the parent's questions about the test.) That's great. How about on this row? Now which circle in this first group looks like a doorbell?" Imitating doorbell chimes adds to the exclusive relationship that you are developing with the patient, and the testing continues until you have completed the test. If the child takes the glasses off, say very seriously, "Oh I don't want you to touch my special equipment. Let's have fun instead," and proceed on to the Worth four-dot testing, getting the red-green glasses on the same way. Some time during this process, I mutter to the parents that I will explain everything I am doing later, once I am through with everything.

Only perform Worth four-dot testing if it is necessary, although it is a great way of demonstrating your mind-reading powers to children. It is easy to not-so-subtly convince them that they better not lie about anything. You know just what they see. As you cover the green eye say, "Now you see two reds, don't you?" and nod your head in an all-knowing, positive, authoritative way.

In order to complete Worth four-dot testing on a very young child, I invite the child to touch the lights while I count. In an attempt to get positive answers, I ask an older child, "Do you see some lights? Any red ones? How many?" The key question if the patient claims to see five lights is to differentiate between diplopia (and what kind of diplopia) and rapid alternation. "Do you see reds and greens at the same time, or first one, then the other?" I still have not made eye contact with the parent as I mutter, "No, this isn't a color vision test." Hopefully by now, the parent should realize he or she merely provides a lap for the child thus keeping interruptions to a minimum. Table 2-3 indicates the possible response and method for recording Worth four-dot testing. The Worth four-dot test is performed at near (one-third of a meter), which tests more peripherally, and at distance (6 meters), which tests more centrally.

Haploscopic devices are not readily available in most offices. These instruments, such as the synoptophore or troposcope, allow each eye to be presented with a different target so that assessment of the patient's retinal correspondence and sensory and motor fusion can be made.

Motor fusion is tested when control of the patient's alignment is assessed. It is, therefore, covered in the next section.

Part 3. Alignment

A patient's strabismic deviation has three components: control, direction, and size.

Control

Control is tested by the cover–uncover test. This is generally done during a routine eye exam by the single cover test, which determines the presence of a phoria, tropia, or intermittent tropia. The patient must steadily maintain fixation on a target that requires and stimulates his or her accommodation. Most patients will not accommodate on a fixation light, and therefore, a penlight should not be used for fixation. Many patients will not accommodate on the 20/200 E or on the stuffed dog at the end of the room. To make a patient fixate and accommodate, you must force the patient to attempt to identify small objects. While you perform the cover test, ask the patient, "How many whiskers does the dog have? Is he sitting or walking? Read me the 20/40 line backward. Forward. What letter is above the Z?" This causes the patient to maintain accommodation and fixation while you assess eye alignment. The patient should have a cover–uncover test performed at distance fixation, preferably 20 feet or 6 meters, and at near fixation at 14 inches or one-third meter. As one eye is covered, the opposite eye is observed for movement. As the eye is uncovered, it is observed for movement. Table 2-4 breaks down the possible movement responses when the right eye is cover–uncovered describing a phoria, tropia, or intermittent deviation. Table 2-5 is a similar algorithm for the left eye as it is cover–uncovered.

Vergence amplitudes of a fusing patient are another method of judging control. However, these measurements should not be taken until all other alignment measurements are done. Generally, the examiner would want to determine how well a patient with an exodeviation can converge or how well a patient with an esodeviation can diverge. The horizontal prism bar is gradually introduced starting with the one and moving up to larger prisms using base-In to measure dIvergence, and base-Out to measure cOnvergence. The patient maintains fixation and fusion as the amount of prism is increased and then is instructed to report when diplopia is appreciated. The measurement is performed first at distance and then again at near. Seeing two images is the signal that the vergence amplitude has been exhausted. This is the break point. Reducing the prism until fusion is regained is a signal of the patient's ability to recover fusion and, normally, should be only one or two incremental steps down from the break point. This is the recovery point. While measuring convergence, a patient should also be instructed to report when the single image blurs, as this is a signal of the inappropriate use of accommodative convergence to maintain binocularity. This is the blur point. The patient may be able to converge a lot, but the image is blurry. Their pupils may overconstrict at the moment they overaccommodate and blur. This is a classic finding in patients with symptomatic convergence insufficiency who will complain of blurred vision after a few minutes of reading. The print may never actually double; it just blurs.

Table 2-4

Cover–Uncover Right Eye—Test Requires Central Vision in Each Eye

If, when covering OD:	This means:	If, when uncovering OD:	This means:
1. OS doesn't move	OS was fixing	A. OD doesn't move either	Either ortho or R tropia (confirms with Table 2-5, Step 1)
		B. OD moves in	OD was out—exophoria
		C. OD moves out	OD was in—esophoria
		D. OD moves down	OD was up—hyperphoria or DVD
		E. OD moves up	OD was down—hypophoria
		F. Combination	
2. OS moves in	OS was out (LXT)	A. OD doesn't move now	Alternating XT
		B. OD moves back in to fix	LXT, prefers OD
3. OS moves out	OS was in (LET)	A. OD doesn't move now	Alternating ET
		B. OD moves back out to fix	LET, prefers OD
4. OS moves down	OS was up (LHT)	A. OD doesn't move	LHT, which alternates now
		B. OD moves back up to fix	LHT, prefers OD
5. OS moves up	OS was down (L hypo T)	A. OD doesn't move	RHT, which alternates now
		B. OD moves back down to fix	RHT, prefers OD
6. Combination of moves	Combined horizontal/vertical	A. Combination	
7. OS has unsteady fixation	Latent nystagmus		

DVD = dissociated vertical deviation

Direction

Direction of the strabismus is determined by the direction of movement of the eye during cover measurements. Essentially, an eye that moves out to fixate must have been in (eso) under that cover. An eye that moves in must have been out (exo), up must have been down (hypo), and down must have been up (hyper). Table 2-6 lists the commonly used abbreviations for strabismic deviations.

Size

The size of the existing deviation is measured with prisms. The more sophisticated the test, the more accurate it will be. Table 2-7 lists methods of measuring strabismus from the least sophisticated test to the most sophisticated. While the Maddox rod can give you very accurate measurements, it also has the most limitations and, therefore, should not be used on most patients.

Table 2-5

Cover–Uncover Left Eye—Test Requires Central Vision in Each Eye

If, when covering OS:	This means:	If, when uncovering OS:	This means:
1. OD doesn't move	OD was fixing	A. OS doesn't move either	Either ortho or L tropia (confirm with Table 2-4, Step 1)
		B. OS moves in	OS was out—exophoria
		C. OS moves out	OS was in—esophoria
		D. OS moves down	OS was up—hyperphoria or DVD
		E. OS moves up	OS was down—hypophoria
		F. Combination	
2. OD moves in	OD was out (RXT)	A. OS doesn't move now	Alternating XT
		B. OS moves back in to fix	RXT, prefers OS
3. OD moves out	OD was in (RET)	A. OS doesn't move now	Alternating ET
		B. OS moves back out to fix	RET, prefers OS
4. OD moves downs	OD was up (RHT)	A. OS doesn't move	RHT, which alternates now
		B. OS moves back up to fix	RHT, prefers OS
5. OD moves up	OD was down (R hypo T)	A. OS doesn't move	LHT, which alternates now
		B. OS moves back down to fix	LHT, prefers OS
6. Combination of moves	Combined horizontal/vertical	A. Combination	
7. OD has unsteady fixation	Latent nystagmus		

Table 2-6

Strabismus Abbreviations

Tropia	T
Intermittent tropia, add ()	(T)
Phoria, drop T	
Esodeviation	E
Exodeviation	X
Hyperdeviation, add R or L eye H	RH or LH
Hypodeviation, add R or L hypo	R hypo or L hypo
Dissociated vertical deviation	DVD
Add R or L eye	R DVD or L DVD
Near, add prime'	ET'

Examples:

Left exotropia	LXT
Right hypertropia	RHT
Left dissociated vertical deviation	L DVD
Esophoria at near	E'
Right hypotropia at distance	R hypo T
Intermittent exotropia at near	X(T)'

Table 2-7

Strabismus Measurement Techniques

Least sophisticated

1. Hirschberg
2. Krimsky
3. Prism and cover
4. Maddox rod

Most sophisticated

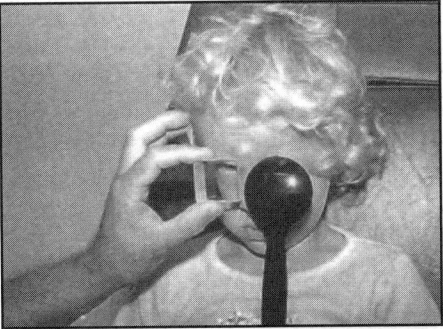
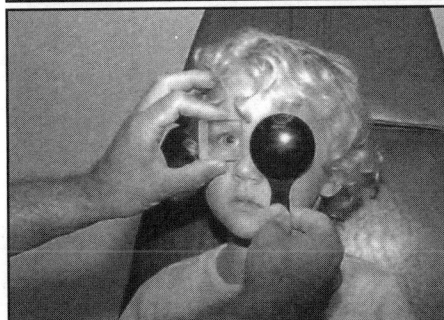
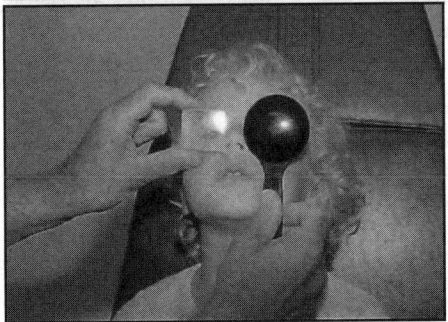

Figure 2-1. The patient is measured in the primary position with the head straight and in up- and downgazes by positioning the head while instructing to fixate on the target.

Done accurately, prism and cover measurements are considered the "gold standard" of measurements.

Size measurements should be performed at distance fixation and at near. The distance measurement should include the straight-ahead, or primary position, plus the secondary positions of up, down, right, and left gazes. Figure 2-1 shows a patient being measured in primary, up, and

Figure 2-2. During head tilt measuring for the 3ST, the base of the prism is held parallel to the floor of the patient's orbit, not parallel to the floor of the room.

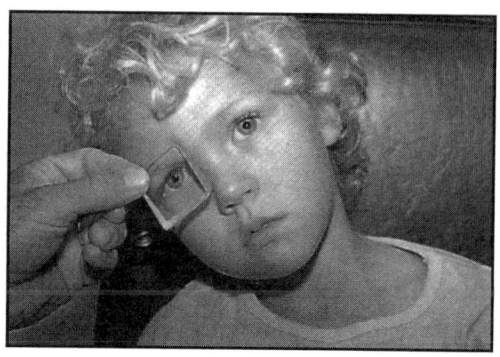

down gazes. The presence of a hyperdeviation requires head tilt measurements. Figure 2-2 shows the correct prism position for the measurement of a hyperdeviation during head tilt measurement. Note the base of the prism is held parallel to the floor of the patient's orbit, not to the floor of the room. Completion of measurements in those fields will yield enough information to determine the presence of incomitance and/or the existence of an A or V pattern. The application of the Three Step Test (3ST) determines which of the eight cyclovertical extraocular muscles is weak; this is covered later in this chapter. Measurements at near should be done in the primary position and in the reading/downgaze position. Any esodeviation should be remeasured with plus lenses (+3.00 typically). Any patient who is almost presbyopic should also be remeasured with plus lenses to see if his or her deviation is significantly changed with his or her impending presbyopic correction.

Subjective Versus Objective Measurements

When first starting out, it is tempting to measure strabismus using only the Maddox rod because it seems so accurate. The patient seems to do all of the work; he or she actually tells you how much his or her deviation is quibbling over if it is 7 or 8 prism diopters (PD) of some kind of eso. But there are some major drawbacks to using the Maddox rod, which is why most strabismus practices rarely use it. As a measurement test, it requires the most of the patient: decent vision, cooperation and willingness to give you the correct answer, and normal retinal correspondence (NRC) even while tropic. See Table 2-8 for requirements for getting accurate measurements dependent on the test. Unfortunately, if you follow the rules and measure stereopsis and determine the patient to be bifoveal, measure Worth four-dot and get a fusion response, and then do the single cover test and get a tropia (which is possible), you do not know if the patient has NRC. Furthermore, one patient can sometimes have NRC and then flip over to abnormal or anomalous retinal correspondence (ARC), which will totally alter your Maddox rod measurements. So my best advice is DO NOT USE the Maddox rod for measuring strabismus. Get comfortable with all of the other methods of measuring that are objective and do not hinge on a patient's retinal correspondence.

Penlights, Fixation, and Accommodation

Whether performing Krimsky with prisms, or Hirschberg and guessing at the tropia you see, one rule must prevail. The penlight that you hold and shine in the patient's eyes is for you to see, not for the patient to look at. The classic descriptions of either test always instruct the patient to

Table 2-8
Measurement Requirements

Test	Vision	Retinal Correspondence	Patient Cooperation	Fixation Distance	Target
Hirschberg	In one eye	Not required	Needs to fixate	Near test	Accommodative
Krimsky	In one eye	Not required	Fixate, prism near face	Near test and distance estimate	Accommodative
Prism and cover	In each eye	Not required	Fixate, prism and cover, near face	Near test and distance test	Accommodative
Maddox rod (MR)	In each eye	Normal	Fixate, prism and MR near face, comprehension	Near test Distance test awkward	Nonaccommodative

"look" at the so-called fixation light; but that is not an accommodative target. You must have a fixation target for the patient to be interested in, whether it is a finger puppet (for a very young child) or your regular fixation stick held adjacent to the viewing light. This will increase the likelihood that accommodation is being exerted by the patient and, therefore, the real measurement will be elicited.

Hirschberg Measurements

Hirschberg measurements assess the relative position of the light reflex in each eye. Usually, if the reflexes are symmetrical, even if not centrally located, the child probably has no eye turn. When the reflexes are asymmetrical, a tropia may exist. The direction of the eye turn is determined by the direction of displacement of the corneal light reflex from the normal position. An eye that deviates INward has a corneal reflex that is displaced OUTward. The amount of eye turn is the number of millimeters of displacement, where 1 mm displacement = 7 degrees = 15 PD (approximately). Considering that a child's pupillary diameter is about 4 mm and the corneal diameter is 12 mm, a light reflex at the pupillary margin indicates a 30 PD turn. A light reflex at the limbus indicates a 90 PD turn (Figure 2-3).

Krimsky Measurements

Krimsky measurements use prisms to artificially place the deviated light reflex onto the appropriate relative position when compared to the fixing eye. When the correcting prism moves the light reflexes so that they match symmetrically, the amount of prism is the amount of tropia measured by the Krimsky method.

A child who fixates with either eye can have the prism placed over either eye. Correcting prisms are placed over the fixing eye in patients having a blind eye that cannot fixate or with young children who strongly prefer one eye. In this way, you know that the eye under the prism is fixing centrally and you are better able to see the light reflex of the nonfixing eye. A base-out

Figure 2-3. Hirschberg measurements: 90 PD LXT—light reflex of the left eye deviates to the nasal limbus (top). 45 PD RET—light reflex of the right eye deviates temporally between the limbus and pupillary border (middle). 30 PD LXT—light reflex of the left eye deviates to the nasal pupillary border (bottom).

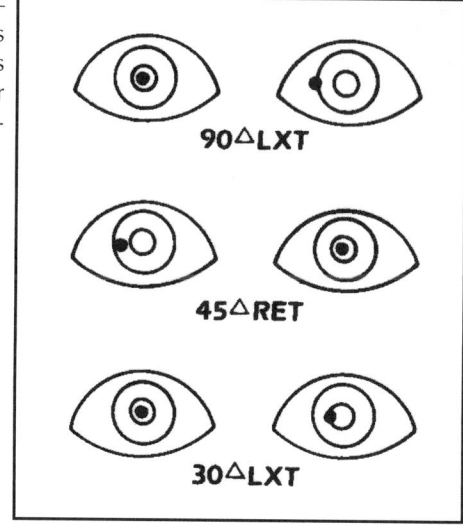

prism is used to correct an esotropia (ET); a base-in prism is used to correct an exotropia (XT). A base-down prism is used to correct a hypertropia, and a base-up prism to correct a hypotropia.

In regard to all measurement tests, remember one rule: eye IN causes the corneal light reflex to be displaced OUT, requires correcting prism base-OUT, and displaces the diplopic image OUT (Figure 2-4).

So if the eye is up, the reflex is down, and you would use base-down prism over that eye to correct it. If you had the Worth four-dot red lens over that eye, the red image would appear displaced downward in a patient with NRC.

Prism and Cover Measurements

Prism and cover measurements (P + C) require steady fixation with either eye and, therefore, may not be as accurate on infants or some very young children. The patient's vision must be good enough to fixate accurately. P + C measurements also require that both eyes move freely, thus it cannot be used on patients with a restrictive strabismus such as Graves' ophthalmopathy. If one eye is restricted, the test must be modified by placing the prism over the restricted "frozen" eye. The patient must fixate on an accommodative target (a 20/40 or smaller letter if he or she sees 20/20) and continue to accommodate on it. Nonaccommodation leads to a major source of error when taking measurements. Instruct the patient to read different lines of letters—backward, forward—and to identify, for example, the third letter of the second line, so that he or she continues to accommodate. Do not instruct patients to simply "look at the E," because once they have seen it (regardless of its size), they can look at it steadily without necessarily accommodating. When this happens, the full deviation does not become manifest, preventing accurate measurement.

The cover is alternately placed over each eye, never allowing binocularity to take place. The direction of the phoria, tropia, or intermittent tropia has been determined by the cover–uncover test, and usually the correcting prism may be placed over either eye. The prism is increased or decreased until no movement of either eye occurs with cross-covering. The use of a larger prism at this point results in reversal of eye movement when cross-covering. Sometimes a patient does not fixate well or steadily and the eyes make an extra back-and-forth movement—a redress movement—each time the cover is moved. Neutralization is then estimated to be when the movement

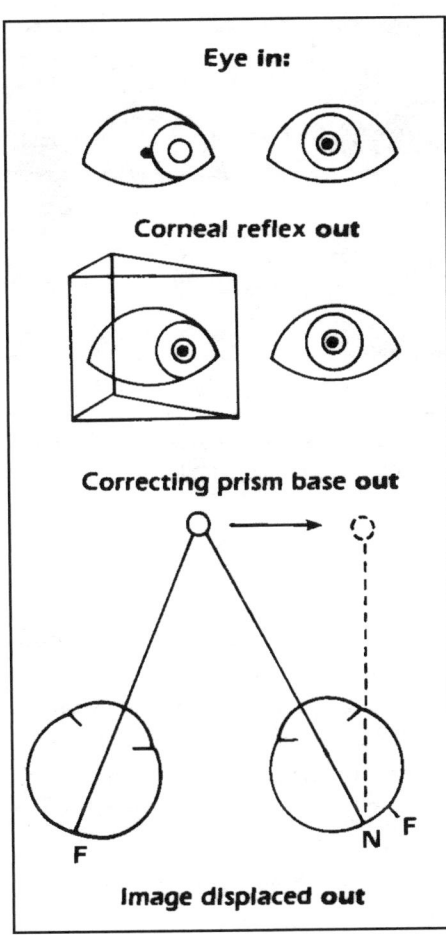

Figure 2-4. Eye in—reflex out, base out, image out.

is an equal amount in each direction. The amount of prism that neutralizes the eye movement is the measured size of deviation.

Occasionally, only one eye will seem to be neutralized with a given prism and the fellow eye will continue to move. This is a tip-off that a primary and secondary deviation exists. A patient who measures the same with either eye fixing will appear to be neutralized when the same strength prism is placed over either eye. When the deviation cannot be neutralized in both eyes by the same prism, you must consciously measure the primary and secondary deviation.

First, cover the left eye so that the right eye is fixing. Place the correcting prism under the cover over the left eye. Then move the cover to the right eye and watch for movement of the left eye under the prism. With the appropriate correcting prism, no movement of the left eye should occur when the cover is moved. Record the deviation with the right eye fixing.

Then measure the deviation with the left eye fixing. Cover the right eye and place the correcting prism under the cover. Move the cover from the right eye to the left and watch for movement of the right eye. This will be the deviation with the left eye fixing. When measurements are to be done with either the right or the left eye fixing by P + C, the correcting prism should be placed in the opposite eye.

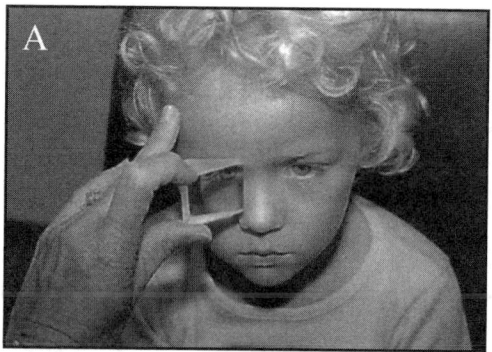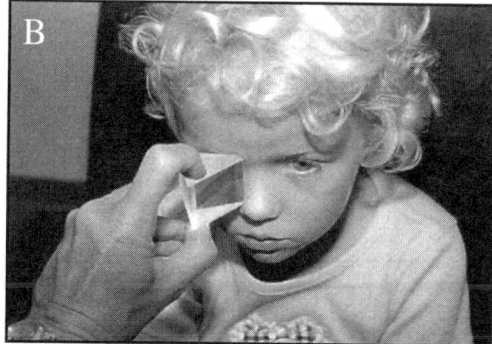

Figure 2-5. (A) The picture shows the proper placement of a right angle plastic prism. Note that the right angle side is parallel to the patient's frontal plane. The base of the prism is then parallel to the patient's line of sight. (B) The picture shows that an isosceles prism is held so that one side of the prism is parallel to the patient's frontal plane. The base of the prism is then not parallel to the patient's line of sight. This is proper placement for plastic prisms.

Simultaneous Prism and Cover Measurements

Another way of measuring a deviation with either eye fixing is by the simultaneous prism and cover test (S P + C). A patient is asked to fixate with one eye, and that eye is covered as the correcting prism is simultaneously placed over the deviating eye. (The cover and prism are simultaneously introduced.) If no movement is perceived, the deviation is neutralized. Typically, the S P + C measurement would be made before the alternate prism and cover measurements and just after the cover–uncover test. Because this method does not involve cross-covering, the S P + C only measures the tropia that is normally manifest and should be done prior to any cross-covering, which would measure the largest deviation possible as well as the size of the phoria.

Extra Tips for Accurate Measurements Using Plastic Prisms

Prisms come in two shapes: right angle (like most prisms 25 diopters [D] or more) and isosceles (like the smaller prisms in the box). The flat side of the right angle prism is placed closer to the patient in his or her frontal plane. Either side of an isosceles prism may be placed in the patient's frontal plane (Figure 2-5).

For deviations larger than 50 PD, split the correcting prisms, never stack them unless measuring a vertical deviation with a horizontal. A vertical prism may be stacked on a horizontal prism. The largest prism available is 50 D. Any time a patient measures more than 50, a second prism must be added to the fellow eye. Always use the 50, then add prism to the second eye until neutralization is reached. Place the smaller prism (the 12) over the fixing eye, which will not be fixing straight ahead by 12 PD worth.[1]

High refractive errors change the actual amount of deviation from the amount traditionally measured with prisms. Tables A-1 and A-2 (in the Appendix) show the adjustments needed to accurately provide measurements on patients with strabismus and high myopia or hyperopia.

Three Step Test

The 3ST is based on the synergistic and antagonistic qualities of pairs of extraocular muscles (EOMs). There are three steps, each of which eliminates half of the remaining potential muscles,

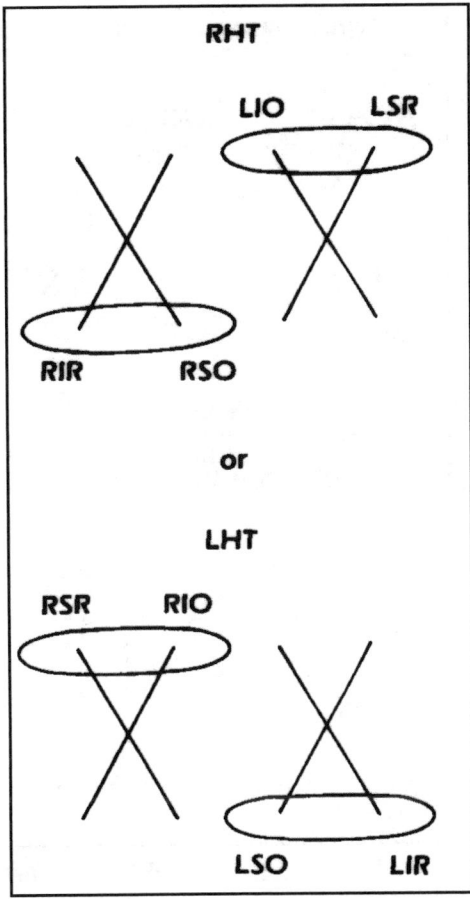

Figure 2-6. The 3ST. Step 1: An RHT could be due to a palsy of the right eye depressors RSO, RIR, or the left eye elevators LIO, LSR. The two muscle pairs are circled to indicate them as possible causes of the incomitant RHT (top). An LHT could be due to a palsy of the right eye elevators RSR, RIO, or the left eye depressors LIR, LSO (bottom).

leaving only one muscle to be blamed after the three steps. The 3ST requires working knowledge of all muscle actions and the position in which each action is best executed.

Step 1—Determine the presence of a right or left hypertropia (RHT or LHT) in the primary position. (If the patient's presenting sign is a hypodeviation, consider it a hyperdeviation of the opposite eye.) An RHT implies that the weak muscle could be one of the right eye depressors (right superior oblique [RSO], right inferior rectus [RIR]) or the left eye elevators (left inferior oblique [LIO], left superior rectus [LSR]) (Figure 2-6). An LHT implies that the weak muscle could be one of the right eye elevators (right inferior oblique [RIO], right superior rectus [RSR]) or the left eye depressors (left superior oblique [LSO], left inferior rectus [LIR]). The two possible muscle pairs are circled in Figure 2-6.

Step 2—Determine if the hypertropia (HT) is larger in right or left gaze. An HT largest in right gaze implies that one of the right gaze vertically acting muscles is weak. (The RSR, RIR work vertically in ABDuction in right gaze; the LIO, LSO work vertically in ADDuction in right gaze [Figure 2-7].) The left gaze vertically acting muscles are the LSR, LIR, RIO, and RSO. Again, the two possible muscle pairs are circled. After Steps 1 and 2, when the circles are superimposed, only two muscles have two circles around them.

After Step 2, only two muscles are left as possible candidates. There is always one from each eye; one is an oblique, the other is a rectus muscle, but both are either superior muscles (intort-

Figure 2-7. The 3ST. Step 2: An HT worse in right gaze is due to a palsy of one of the right gaze verticals—RSR, RIR, LIO, LSO (top). An HT worse in left gaze could be due to a palsy of one of the left gaze verticals—LSR, LIR, RIO, RSO (bottom).

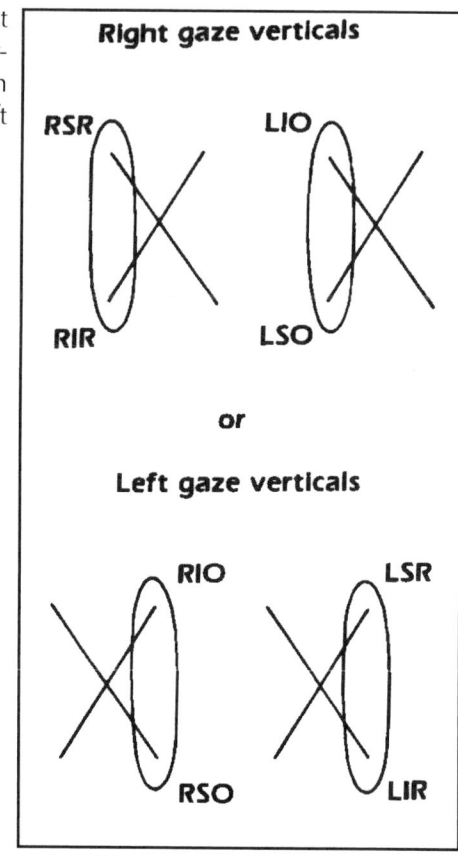

ers) or inferior muscles (extorters). Step 3 will determine which of these two muscles is the weak cyclovertical muscle.

Step 3—Determine if the HT is larger when measured during head tilt to the right or left. Proper measurement requires holding the base of the prism parallel to the floor of the orbit, not parallel to the floor of the room. If Maddox rod is used, it should be held so that the line visible to the patient is parallel to the floor of the orbit. The correcting prism should be positioned so that its base is also parallel to the floor of the orbit (Figure 2-8).

When the patient tilts his or her head to the right, the right eye attempts to right itself by intorting; the left eye tries to extort. The right head tilt torters are the RSR, RSO, LIO, and LIR. The left head tilt torters are the RIO, RIR, LSO, and LSR (Figure 2-9). These two muscle pairs would be circled, leaving only one muscle with three circles around it when the circles are superimposed. This is the palsied muscle.

After Step 2, two intorters or two extorters remain as possibly weak muscles. One is from each eye and only one is being tested during head tilt to the right, while the other is tested during head tilt to the left.

For example, if the RSR and LSO were left after Step 2, both are superior muscles (intorters), one is a rectus, the other an oblique, and one is from each eye. During head tilt to the right, only the intorters of the right eye are innervated. If the RSR was the palsied muscle, its synergist for intorsion, the RSO, would help intort. The RSO is also a depressor, and working to depress the

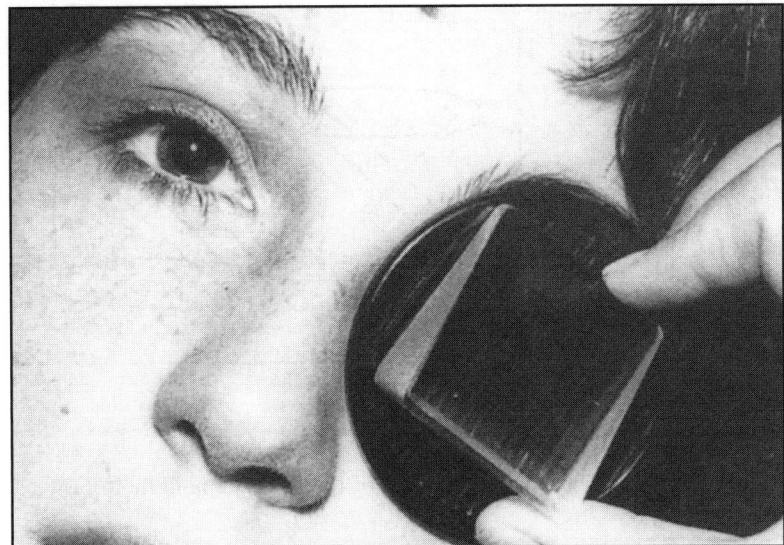

Figure 2-8. The 3ST. Maddox rod measurements of a patient with LHT. Head is tilted to the left and the base of the prism is held parallel to the floor of the orbit. The Maddox rod is held so that the red line (visible to the patient) is also parallel to the floor of the orbit.

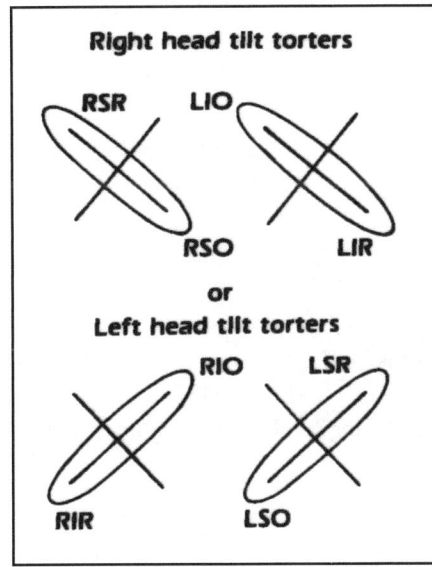

Figure 2-9. The 3ST. Step 3: An HT worse on right head tilt could be due to a palsy of the right eye intorters—RSR or RSO, or the left eye extorters—LIO or LIR (top). An HT worse on left head tilt could be due to a palsy of one of the right eye extorters—RIR or RIO, or the left eye intorters—LSO or LSR (bottom).

eye against a weak RSR would result in the eye dropping hypo. Thus, the original LHT would be largest during head tilt to the right in an RSR palsy.

If the LSO was palsied instead, it would try to intort the eye only during head tilt to the left. Its synergist for intorsion, the LSR, would also be elevating the left eye against a weak LSO (which should normally be depressing the eye). Therefore, a weak LSO would result in an increased LHT during head tilt to the left.

Figure 2-10. Cyclovertical muscle pairs implied by the 3ST in an RIO palsy.

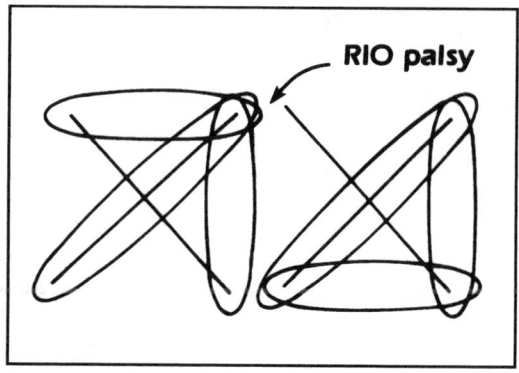

RIO palsy

The Three Step Test in Practice

Circle the pairs of muscles potentially at fault after each of the three steps in the following examples:

Example:

Step 1—LHT

Step 2—Worse in left gaze

Step 3—Worse in left tilt

Step 1 leaves LSO, LIR, RIO, or RSR as possibly weak

Step 2 leaves LIR or RIO as still possible weak

Step 3 leaves RIO weak because the right eye extorts during left head tilt (Figure 2-10)

Example:

Step 1—RHT

Step 2—Worse in right gaze

Step 3—Worse in left tilt

Step 1 leaves RSO, RIR, LIO, or LSR as possibly weak

Step 2 leaves RIR or LIO as still possibly weak

Step 3 leaves RIR weak because the right eye extorts during left head tilt (Figure 2-11)

Example:

Step 1—Small RHT, nearly ortho

Step 2—RHT worse in left gaze, but LHT worse in right gaze

Step 3—RHT worse in right tilt, but LHT worse in left tilt

This last example is a special 3ST problem. It is a classic example of a bilateral SO palsy, a fairly common finding following head trauma. Although there may be almost no deviation in the primary position, there is usually a large V pattern ET and RHT in left gaze and LHT in right gaze. The patient may also complain of torsional diplopia, as bilateral SO palsies often result in more than 10 degrees of extorsion. To make the 3ST work in this situation, consider the RHT by itself (Step 1—RHT, Step 2—RHT worse in left gaze, Step 3—RHT worse in right head tilt), which will indicate an RSO palsy. Then consider the LHT by itself (Step 1—LHT, Step 2—LHT worse in right gaze, Step 3—LHT worse in left head tilt), which will indicate an LSO palsy (Figure 2-12).

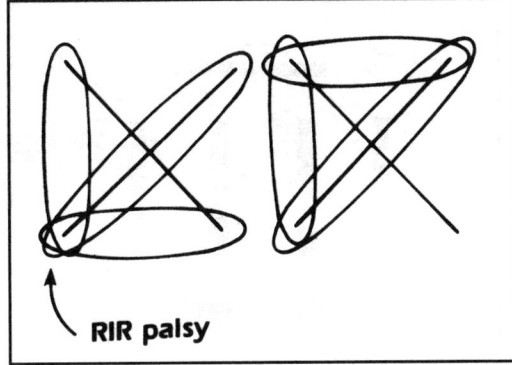

Figure 2-11. Cyclovertical muscle pairs implied by the 3ST in an RIR palsy.

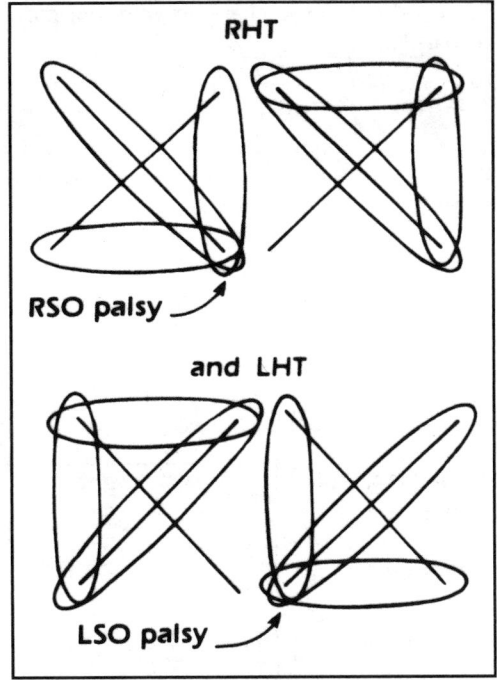

Figure 2-12. Cyclovertical muscle pairs implied by the 3ST in a bilateral SO palsy—RSO palsy (top), LSO palsy (bottom).

Measuring Dissociated Vertical Deviation

Dissociated vertical deviation (DVD) is a type of vertical deviation that both defies good explanation and eludes straightforward measurements. Either eye will elevate under cover occlusion, yet a DVD does not behave as a hyperphoria/tropia. In a DVD, the eye that is not elevated never drops below the midline. Most DVDs are asymmetrical with one eye elevating more than the other when it is occluded under the cover. A DVD may appear to be unilateral, a situation that is distinguished from a hyperphoria/tropia because the eye that does not elevate under cover occlusion (the non-DVD eye) also never drops hypotropic (below the midline) when the DVD eye fixates.

Measurement of the DVD is done in two steps: right eye then left eye. Base-down prism is placed before the right eye, and the P + C measurement is made. The prismed right eye is the only one watched by the examiner, and the occluder is held over the right eye for several seconds during each cross-cover. The prism's strength is increased while the occluder is kept over the right eye so that fusion is never allowed during the entire measurement process. Neutralization occurs when no downward movement of the right eye is perceived while moving the cover from the prismed right eye over to the left eye. The key to obtaining the full DVD measurement is to allow the occluder to remain over the prismed deviating eye for several seconds longer than usual, as the DVD often takes several seconds longer to dissociate than a phoric or tropic eye does.

The second step is to measure the left eye with the correcting base-down prism over the left eye, the occluder lingering over the left eye, and the examiner only watching the movement of the left eye.

Figure 2-13. A single character with four crowding bars.

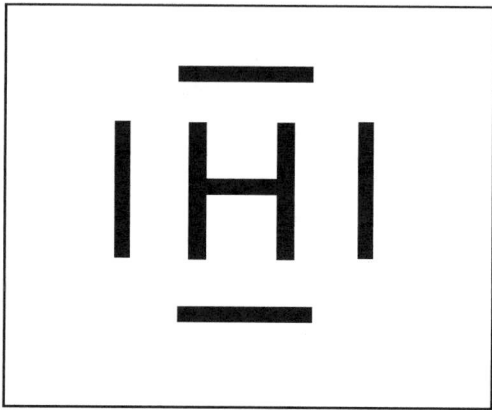

Figure 2-14. Three Allen picture cards held together to elicit crowding phenomenon.

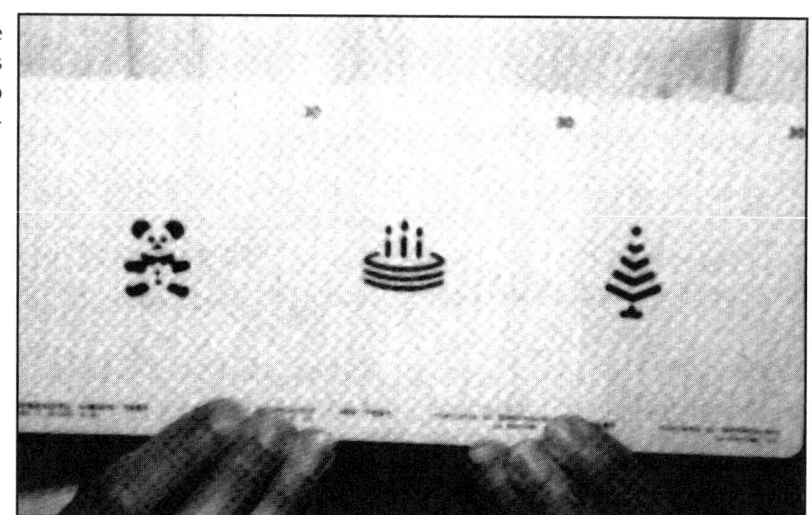

Part 4. Vision Testing, LAST

Vision testing on young children is essential in order to determine decreased vision caused by uncorrected refractive error or ocular pathology and to diagnose amblyopia, one of the major causes of poor vision in children. Amblyopia is poor vision in the brain, even though the correct glasses lens may be in place. Amblyopia can be corrected only prior to visual maturity, so the diagnosis must be made before visual maturity occurs. Therefore, you are committed to taking an accurate monocular vision on every child you have before you.

Since amblyopic eyes are more sensitively tested when a full line of character optotypes (test figures) are displayed, showing the child one picture or one letter at a time is precisely the wrong thing to do. The alternative to this is using crowded single optotypes that display the single character with four bars around it to simulate a full line of symbols (Figure 2-13). Children do find it easier to report single characters rather than a full line of characters, and the Allen picture cards have remained in offices for years, but if you are checking a child, you are checking for amblyopia. If you are checking for amblyopia, then you must show a full line of optotypes, or ones that have the crowding bars. Figure 2-14 illustrates a suitable method for Allen picture testing when only the cards are available.

Table 2-9

Vision Tests

Most sophisticated

1. ETDRS
2. Snellen
3. Crowded HOTV or Lea symbols
4. Allen pictures (held together)*
5. Teller acuity cards
6. Fix and follow
7. Central, steady, maintained (CSM)

Least sophisticated

Rarely used in pediatric ophthalmology practices

Table 2-9 lists the available vision tests in order of most sophisticated to least. The electronically generated ETDRS vision system shows single but crowded Snellen style letters in a system that scores vision by repeatedly crossing the threshold of vision. The score is translated into a Snellen style vision. When a Snellen line is used for a child, the vision is scored as for adults, recording the smallest line that is perceived accurately. If the patient sees all of the 20/25 line clearly, but only two of the letters on the 20/20 line, then the vision is recorded as 20/25 + 2.

Vision should be recorded for each eye, with correction, at distance and near.

Determine for yourself what test children will be capable of performing accurately before the patch goes on. If you do not, you will have no idea that they cannot call out the Snellen letters because they cannot see, are distracted by the patch, distracted by a sibling, or because they just do not know their letters as well as their mother boasts.

The key to accurate vision testing is good occlusion of the eye not being tested. The best way to ensure proper occlusion is with an adhesive patch placed on the skin under any glasses. Obviously, putting the patch on the child can be a challenge, and I use this approach (after completion of the alignment measurements). To get my patch on the eye with the least commotion, I open the package and answer any questions about, "What is that?" with, "I'll show you....feel this," and I invite the child to touch the soft lining part, as I say, "This is very soft, and grey, just like my cat at home. This is so soft I can put it right here (as I place it on the child's eye) and it won't bother you. It doesn't hurt. But it feels a little funny though, doesn't it?" I purposely put the patch on lightly so that it can be removed easily and switched to the second eye without hurting the skin. Of course, barely sticking the patch on only works if the child is not allowed to touch it. It is essential that the child not touch the patch since it is mine, and I tell him or her that it might be impossible for me to get it off if he or she has touched it. If the child is young, I tell the parent to hold the child's hands, give him or her a big hug, and not to let go as I put the patch on.

Being the first person to physically put a patch onto a young child who might be amblyopic is a huge opportunity to introduce the idea of wearing a patch to both parent and child. It is certainly worthwhile to take a few moments to ensure that the adults will prevail during vision testing. It also sets the parents up for success if they are directed to patch the child at home, use glasses, or use drops.

Typically, I would test the right eye first: distance vision, near vision, perform retinoscopy, recheck vision with any significant refractive error, then repeat for the left eye. Again, moving quickly from one test to another is essential to perform a successful exam on a young child.

Additional objective vision tests are helpful in young children. Tests such as fix and follow, or central, steady, and maintained done monocularly do not require excellent vision and are therefore less likely to accurately diagnose amblyopia. They are helpful, however, in determining the presence of vision in a child suspected of not seeing. A brightly lit finger puppet will elicit fix and follow movements despite very poor vision. Resist the parents' offer to help you by handing you their jangling car keys to use as a test object. You are testing vision, not hearing.

Tropia tests determine which eye is preferred when the child is given a choice of fixating with either eye. This choice happens naturally with a tropic deviation or an intermittent one that can be broken down. The preference for fixing with one eye indicates poorer vision in the non-preferred eye.

When the eyes are straight, a tropia can be induced with prisms. A 10 diopter vertical prism will cause a child with equal vision to alternate fixation up and down. A 25 diopter base-in prism will cause a child with equal vision to fixate with the eye without the prism. Repeating the test with the prism over the other eye will confirm that either the child plainly alternates or prefers to look with the eye without the prism, which would indicate equal vision. Amblyopia would be strongly suspected in a child who preferred to consistently look with one eye despite the large prism over it.

Pupils are the final test performed; dazzling the retina now will not matter since the fusion, alignment, and vision have all been assessed.

So now your basic four-part exam, including history, fusion, alignment, and vision, is complete. Understanding the different types of strabismus problems will help you know what additional tests are needed to confirm the diagnosis and assist in making the treatment plan.

Reference

1. Hansen VC. Common pitfalls in measuring strabismic patients. *Am Orthopt J*. 1989;393:3-11.

Chapter 3

Approaching Children and Infants

KEY POINTS

- Vision screening is the most important step in detecting amblyopia and other vision and alignment problems in children.

- Children with reading/learning problems must have an eye examination.

- Patients with untreatable amblyopia should wear safety eyewear at all times for the rest of their lives.

What makes examining children and infants so unique? An accurate eye exam requires a certain amount of cooperation on the part of the child. No one—child, parent, or examiner—wants to resort to forcibly holding down a patient in order to obtain information. Everyone wants the ophthalmic experience to go successfully, as smoothly as possible, and hopefully, with an element of fun.

The essence of the examination of a young child or infant is speed, as covered in Chapter 2. The best advice about learning to take strabismus measurements is to practice on cooperative adults before attempting them on that moving 2-year-old target.

Besides the potential for being uncooperative, what makes the examination of infants and young children different from that of adults is that the child's visual system is immature. This makes children susceptible to amblyopia and permanent loss of their fusional abilities. When amblyopia is detected early, by the age of 3 to 4 years, recovery of the child's vision is more likely to be successful. When amblyopia is detected well after the age of visual maturity, or after 9 years of age, treatment is less likely to improve vision. Recent multicenter studies on amblyopia conducted by the Pediatric Eye Disease Investigator Group of the National Institutes of Health have changed clinicians' thinking of amblyopia and its treatment by providing evidence-based medicine regarding length of prescribed patching, alternatively using atropine, and how old a patient may be and still improve vision with amblyopic treatment. While amblyopia cannot be prevented, early detection leads to its successful treatment. When strabismus is detected early (remember that an infant's eyes should be straight by 4 months of age), the chance of re-establishing some form of binocularity is much greater.

Amblyopia

What makes amblyopia so unique in the pediatric population is that, if left untreated, it is one of the major causes of blindness in the adult population. The treatment is not harsh; glasses alone may successfully treat it. Additional occlusion therapy of the better-seeing eye with an adhesive patch, atropine drops penalization, or Bangerter foil occlusion in combination with near activity work such as coloring or reading is often all that is required for successful treatment. The success rate is high if the amblyopia is detected by age 3 or 4 and has been shown to be still quite successful if initiated at older ages. Studies have shown that teenagers are worth treating because some older children will have a significant improvement in their vision. So while early detection is critical to success, appropriate treatment is the key to success. Vision screening programs are generally carried out by pediatric offices, preschools, and school systems.

Amblyopia is defined as decreased vision in one eye (though it sometimes occurs in both eyes) that cannot be attributed to a specific organic problem and cannot be improved with corrective lenses. It is like suppression that persists under monocular conditions.

Amblyopia may be categorized in several ways. It may be considered functional (which implies that it is treatable) or organic. Organic amblyopia is considered an amblyopia because the actual organic problem is undetectable; the eye seems normal except for decreased vision, which does not improve with appropriate treatment. An amblyopic eye that is functional would improve with appropriate treatment.

The functional amblyopias are named for their different causes. Nonalternating strabismus is both a cause of amblyopia and a sign that amblyopia exists. Sometimes it is difficult to determine which came first. Nonalternating strabismus causes strabismic amblyopia. This type results when the nonpreferred eye is suppressed and does not develop visually. Strabismic amblyopia is fairly common in accommodative esotropias, in which there is frequently a preferred eye. Purely strabismic amblyopia is treated by occlusion of the preferred eye until absolutely equal vision is achieved.

Anisometropic amblyopia occurs when each eye has a different uncorrected refractive error. As a result, only one eye may see clearly at a time. Most often, an anisometropic child with no myopia never uses the more hyperopic eye. Therefore, amblyopia develops in the more hyperopic eye. Whether looking at distance or near, the child will choose to fixate with the eye requiring the lesser accommodation (ie, the less hyperopic eye). A fully balanced correction of the refractive difference between the two eyes is prescribed. Occlusion treatment may still be necessary. An anisometropic child with myopia in one eye often uses that eye for near fixation. Then the less myopic, plano, or hyperopic eye is used for distance fixation. Amblyopia may not occur in these children. They do lack fusion, however, because both eyes cannot see clear images at the same time. A balanced correction would correct this.

Refractive amblyopia results from uncorrected high refractive errors and is characterized by poor visual development in both eyes (possibly asymmetrical). High hyperopes and extreme myopes may develop bilateral refractive amblyopia. Children with uncorrected high astigmatism may develop meridional amblyopia. In this case, part of the retina receives a clearer image while a band of retina 90 degrees away receives a blurred image due to the uncorrected astigmatism. As a result, a band of amblyopia develops in the part of the retina that corresponds to the cylinder axis. Treatment requires full correction of the astigmatism with balancing of the refractive error, and then occlusive therapy, if necessary.

Amblyopia of disuse (amblyopia ex anopsia) results from disuse of the eye once the initial cause of disuse is removed. Examples are congenital ptosis (where the lid consistently covers the visual axis), congenital cataract, retinal hemorrhage, and hyphema. These maladies cause decreased vision, but once they are removed or resolved, amblyopia may persist because of the length of time the eye spent in "disuse," causing the immature eye to stop developing vision. Treatment consists of occlusive treatment of the better eye, with full optical correction as needed.

Esotropia

Two main types of real esotropia (ET) affect children: infantile and accommodative. The first step in making a diagnosis and treatment plan for ET is to eliminate pseudo-ET. This is caused by a flat nasal bridge and epicanthal folds, which give the baby the appearance of having crossed eyes. Pseudo-ET is diagnosed by determining that the infant has straight eyes on the cross-cover test. The Hirschberg light reflex test is much less accurate and can easily miss smaller amounts of strabismus. Additionally, measurement of stereopsis or divergence amplitudes heightens the likelihood of pseudo-ET. Demonstration of full abduction in the absence of obvious lid fissure changes is essential to rule out a VI nerve palsy.

Infantile Esotropia

Infantile ET is characterized by a large ET (often 40 prism diopters [PD] or more) present within the first 6 months of life that persists after 4 months of life, without a significant accommodative component or hyperopic refractive error. Amblyopia is uncommon, due to cross-fixation in which the baby avoids abducting either eye and uses the right eye to view objects to the

Figure 3-1. The bifocal line should be high enough to bisect the pupil when the glasses are in their normally worn position and the patient looks straight ahead. The proper height ensures that a child who is being treated for a high accommodative convergence/accommodation ratio (AC/A) will use the bifocal segment for all near work.

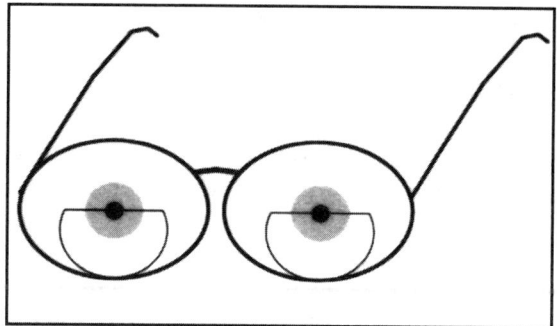

left and the left eye to view objects to the right. V patterns with overactive inferior obliques (IOs) are common, as is DVD. Latent nystagmus is also a frequent finding in patients with infantile ET. The treatment is surgical.

Accommodative Esotropia

Careful control of accommodation is necessary for accurate measurements of all strabismus but particularly of accommodative ET. This is accomplished by continually asking the child to describe fine details about the object that he or she is viewing. Prism and cover (P + C) measurements in the primary and secondary positions at distance and in the primary and downgaze positions at near are necessary during the initial work-up. Additional measurements (uncyclopleged) with plus lenses approximating the cycloplegic refraction should be made at distance and near, and with additional plus at near, if the ET still persists at near despite the approximate cycloplegic refraction. This information will help determine if a bifocal add is necessary.

Accommodative ET classically starts between the ages of 18 months and 3 years and begins as an intermittent eye turn when the child concentrates on something. Occasionally, a child under age 1 will present with accommodative ET, which will need to be distinguished from infantile ET, as treatment is completely different and generally nonsurgical. Older children may develop accommodative ET, sometimes precipitated by a physical or emotional trauma or illness. A new onset ET in an older child, even one that is presumed to be accommodative esotropia, must be distinguished from a neurological process and requires medical decision making.

Cycloplegia must be full, completely reducing the ability to focus and accommodate during cycloplegic refractions. On return visits, check the glasses to make sure the prescription is accurate as well as the fit of the bifocal. Unlike bifocals in adults, the child's bifocal segment line should be high enough so that it bisects the pupil, thus forcing the eyes to look through the bifocal segment for everything held in the hands or in front of the child. The distance segment is only for viewing objects farther than one-third of a meter away (Figure 3-1).

Exotropia

Exotropia (XT) in an infant may be a sign of blindness in one eye. An eye that does not see has no fusional mechanism to help it stay straight, and the eye may drift out. Constant XT in one eye that does not alternate is typically a sign of decreased vision. Many different things could cause the decreased vision, and these are listed in Table 3-1. Remember that monocular blindness could cause an ET, XT, or no strabismus at all.

Table 3-1
Causes of Monocular Blindness in Infancy

- Congenital cataract
- Persistent hyperplastic primary vitreous (PHPV)
- Leukocoria
- Optic nerve hypoplasia
- Tumor: Retinoblastoma
          Rhabdomyosarcoma
- Birth trauma to eye: Hyphema
- Retinal detachment (RD)
- Hemorrhage
- Extreme anisometropia

Other more common forms of XT (phoria, intermittent tropia, constant tropia) may affect patients of any age. XT will be covered in greater detail in Chapter 4.

Torticollis—Head Positioning

Children may mask their eye problem with the use of head positioning. With an abnormal head position, the strabismus or nystagmus may not be evident at all. The easiest way to determine if the head position is hiding something is to gently move the child's head into the opposite position while closely watching the child's eyes, looking for a change in alignment or for nystagmus. If the child continually holds the chin up, encourage the child to look at something fun and move the head down. Occluding one eye should, but may not, eliminate the abnormal head position if it is caused by strabismus. Torticollis may also be an attempt to achieve a pinhole effect to see better with high refractive errors. Children with bilateral high uncorrected hyperopia may use a chin down position, which persists monocularly.

Brown Syndrome—Superior Oblique Tendon Sheath Syndrome

Brown syndrome is manifested by the eye's inability to look up in the adducted position. It is usually a congenital finding but can occasionally be caused by direct trauma or arthritis. Even in previously undiagnosed arthritis, the cartilaginous trochlea may be inflamed, as any joint might be, causing the syndrome.

Reading/Learning Problems

The pediatric ophthalmologist and orthoptist are frequently asked to examine children who have learning difficulties. A tremendous amount of emphasis has been placed on the connection between the eyes, the brain, and learning, although this connection is not always clear. Many visually impaired students are exemplary, while their perfectly sighted counterparts are struggling. The current policy statement entitled *Learning Disabilities, Dyslexia, and Vision*—endorsed by the American Academy of Pediatrics, the American Association for Pediatric Ophthalmology and

Strabismus, and the American Academy of Ophthalmology—states: "There is no known eye or visual cause for dyslexia and learning disabilities and no effective visual treatment." The statement goes on to say that the endorsing groups "strongly support the need for early diagnosis and the need for educational remediation."

However, it is essential that a child with learning difficulties have all the tools necessary to learn. The child's eyes need to be "perfect"; small refractive errors that would not impede the excellent student might be enough to really hinder the struggling student. Latent hyperopia may not be obvious at a standard screening because the child can momentarily make out 20/20 in each eye. Some screening protocols retest distance vision with +3 lenses to detect possible latent hyperopia. Convergence insufficiency may certainly exacerbate reading problems. For these reasons, all children with reading/learning problems should have an eye exam.

Symptoms of convergence insufficiency may include headache, blurring, double vision, eye strain, fatigue while reading, poor concentration, poor recall, and slow reading. Obviously, if this much about the act of looking at a written page and deciphering what it means bothers the child, a dislike of reading could develop. So convergence insufficiency must be ruled out in these children and treated when found. The parents must clearly understand that excellent convergence probably will not make their child a stellar student and reader, but it will not impede his or her progress. Accommodative infacility is rare but may be noted in these students, and plus lenses may help them significantly.

Accommodative effort syndrome is the result of accommodating too much, causing pseudomyopia with subsequent blurring in the distance and excessive crossing while reading. Treatment is aimed at reducing the need to accommodate so excessively.

Functional Amblyopia—Malingering

We see her all the time: 8 years old, failed the school eye exam, wants glasses, and has no refractive error. Malingering is a common finding in the pediatric population, affecting more girls than boys, typically in the 8- to 9-year-old range.[1] Unlike an adult who is almost always looking for monetary gain, a child is just looking for attention or for glasses and the accompanying attention he or she would get. It may have started with an innocent comment like, "I can't always see the blackboard," which was rewarded with a swift response of near hysteria on the parent's/ teacher's part and a quick removal from school to visit the doctor's office. She cannot back down now; the child squints and scrunches, feigns pain when reading the letters, and intuitively stops cold turkey at an average of 20/80 in each eye (distance and near). The pinhole does not help; she has gone blind. When I am the examiner and the exam has gone in this direction, this is what I do. After retinoscopy (which of course yields nearly plano), I confidently explain that I am sure this (−0.12 sphere) lens will help; now read me that line. Painful as it is, T Z V E C L squeaks out. I would never accuse the child of lying because she is not. She is asking for some attention, and she sure got it. Further questioning of the parents (alone) usually yields plenty of explanation, such as the sister got glasses, best friend got glasses, new teacher gives more homework, parents are getting divorced, Grandpa died, etc. Instead of being angry or embarrassed, parents are usually relieved that their child does not have a vision problem, or worse yet, a brain tumor.

Children who are ultimately diagnosed as malingerers may have come into your office innocently enough having failed a school eye exam. During the exam, the typical tip-off that something is wrong is that your findings just do not add up. For instance, such children might have perfect stereopsis but claim 20/400 vision in each eye at near. When doing color testing, they

Table 3-2

Tests for Malingering	Typical Response
Color test plates	Cannot identify
4 diopter prism base-out	No suppression
Retinoscopy measurement	Plano to mild refractive error, but vision improves dramatically*
Stereopsis	Appreciates 40 seconds but claims poor vision (or gets all nine wrong)
Teller acuity cards	Appreciates gratings compatible with 20/20 or gets every presentation wrong (only 50% wrong would be normal if gratings were not seen!)

*It is absolutely necessary to document that each eye was 20/20, even with -0.12 sphere.

cannot even see the test plates. The pinhole does not improve their vision. Have they been hiding in the house, or are they still confidently riding their bike and trotting off to the school bus? These children are so pleased to be left off the hook and told that actually their vision should be just fine, that they do, in fact, get cured. Without directly prompting the child, it will become obvious to the family that their child's vision is fine. Reassurance that they are okay and that they have not done anything bad is the key. Table 3-2 lists some additional tests (and their results) that will help diagnose malingering.

Refractive Errors and Glasses

Refractive measurements are the mainstay of the ophthalmic exam. How are they different in a child? Since visual maturity occurs at around age 9, uncorrected refractive errors can cause amblyopia. Correcting the error with glasses is the first step in treating amblyopia, along with occlusive treatment. It is imperative that the prescription is balanced to allow the exact same amount of accommodating to yield a clear image for each eye. For example, if a cycloplegic refraction yields OD (right eye) +4.50 sphere, OS (left eye) +1.25 + 0.50 X 180, it may not be necessary to fully correct the hyperopia in the left, nonamblyopic eye. A prescription may be given that balances the two eyes by taking 1.25 D from the spherical power of each eye so that OD would be +3.25 sphere and OS PL + 0.50 X 180. The patient would still need to accommodate 1.25 D in each eye to achieve the clearest vision at distance. Full correction of their astigmatic error will put the clearest image on to the retina. Children do not need to have that astigmatic error lessened so that they will "tolerate" it.

Accommodative ET, with or without a high AC/A ratio, is caused by uncorrected hyperopia. Correction of the refractive error eliminates the need to accommodate and, therefore, the need to cross in. Full cycloplegic correction is prescribed, and a bifocal is given if the near ET is greater than the distance measurement. The bifocal segment line should be high enough to bisect the pupil.

Children's glasses should be purchased to wear now, not to grow into. Parents should be warned that, at best, the glasses will fit the child for up to 12 months on average. Like shoes, a very young child will outgrow the frame sooner. The frame style should be such that the child looks through the lens near the geometric center of the lens. Antireflective coating is difficult to keep clean in a child, and unlikely to be appreciated by a child. Scratch coating is not likely to save the lenses from the kind of scratches a child incurs. A better investment is some type of replacement warranty in the event that the frame is broken or the lenses are scratched. (See Chapter 9 for more information about choosing an optical shop.) A child with untreatable amblyopia should be in safety eyewear at all times.

Examining children is both challenging and rewarding. It is up to the examiner to make it fun.

Reference

1. Hansen VC. What do you tell parents about why their child is pretending not to see? *Am Orthopt J.* 2002;52(1):23-30.

Chapter 4

Approaching Adults

KEY POINTS

- Sudden onset diplopia in an adult may be the first sign of systemic disease.

- Indiscriminately dispensing prism to adults may eventually make the condition worse.

Why do orthoptists and pediatric ophthalmologists also specialize in adult strabismus? It is easy to understand once you realize how many pediatric eye problems are actually strabismic. However, approaching an adult with strabismus is nothing like approaching the child with strabismus. Adult eyes are not just bigger versions of children's eyes. It is the brain of the adult with a mature visual system that makes this approach different.

Adults' concerns are different than those of a child (or the child's parents). They may have high unattainable expectations or assume that nothing can be done for them because that is what they have been told before. Adults may be motivated by their visual inability to work or perform the tasks they enjoy like reading or driving. So they may be willing to try anything—prisms, exercises, or more surgery.

Adults may have bad memories of their own childhood experiences at the eye doctor. They remember being patched in a classroom full of normal children. They remember those "one style fits all" frames that patients over 40 have hidden in a drawer somewhere. Not many years ago, insurance companies permitted an overnight stay in the hospital, but usually without their parents, for strabismus surgery. Their eyes may have been patched. They often had discomfort both from the surgery (typically a more painful resection of a rectus muscle combined with its antagonist's recession) and from the use of inferior suture material. They remember throwing up.

All of these things may affect their attitude toward their own eye care. Unfortunately, some adults' memories contribute to their not seeking ophthalmologic care, even for their own children.

All adults are visually mature. Of course, this can be the clinician's friend or enemy. Visual maturity allows an adult to use a compensatory head position in order to regain fusion after a muscle palsy. It allows a patient with a residual eye deviation to attempt to fuse using motor fusion reserves. It also makes the adult who is unable to fuse completely miserable. Visual maturity can also cause an adult to be diplopic after a simple surgery to correct childhood strabismus. An accurate history and examination on adults with strabismus help treat the patient appropriately.

History Taking on Adults With Strabismus

All of the regular rules for history taking still apply to the adult with strabismus. These would include the onset, symptoms, duration, and decompensation. These typical questions are listed in Table 4-1. In addition to those questions, some additional information will help diagnose and treat the adult patient with strabismus.

Is the patient's problem cosmetic or symptomatic? In a world where "looks are everything," patients with strabismus may have been unfairly judged. They may be desperate to change their eye alignment. At the same time, the notion of cosmetic surgery seems like a ridiculous luxury. Strabismus surgery is not in the same billing category as refractive surgery or face lifts, as some patients fear. It is, in fact, usually covered by their insurance because it so often restores binocularity, enhances visual potential, and is reconstructive. Asking, "Do other people notice your eye alignment?" or "Does it bother you that other people can tell that your eyes aren't straight?" usually elicits how patients cosmetically feel about their eyes. Their response is often, "Yes, the people I work with comment that they cannot tell if I'm looking at them or not," or, "Family members notice it getting worse." (Anecdotally, family members frequently claim to have no idea that their loved one has anything wrong with him or her. Of course, they are usually enthusiastic after the surgery but even then will still say they did not see anything wrong before.)

Table 4-1
Adult Strabismus History Questions

Is the patient's complaint visual or cosmetic?

Visual history questions:

Diplopia: Monocular or binocular?

    Ask: If you cover the right eye, does the double vision go away? If you then cover only the left eye, does the double vision go away? (Binocular diplopia exists if the patient answered yes to both questions. Monocular diplopia exists if the double vision persists with one eye covered.)

If binocular diplopia:

    Ask: When did it start? Is it getting better or worse? Were there any precipitating factors: illness, trauma, disease? What makes it worse/better? Are the images horizontal, vertical, torsional, or combination? Are your glasses different or new? (Check for new prism or forgotten prism.)

Eye strain, pain, headache:

    Ask: When? After what visual task? What jobs do you do with your eyes? Do you wake up with it? (Probably not visual.)

Blurry:

    Ask: Same as above. Also: Does the blurring come and go, like a camera going in and out of focus? Do you ever see double? What happens if you only use one eye? (May not be binocularly related.)

Table 4-2
Adult Expectations

- To be symptom-free
- To be symptom-free for most tasks
- To have better cosmesis at the conversational (3 to 5 ft) distance
- To look like he or she did before
- To be able to read comfortably
- To be able to drive safely
- To get rid of prism in glasses
- To be able to wear contact lenses

In symptomatic strabismus, the patient is frequently desperate to be symptom-free, or at least visually comfortable for most of his or her visual tasks. Besides the typical questions listed in Table 4-1, it is also useful to find out what has been tried before as a way of determining what the patient expects can be done now. The range of patient expectations is listed in Table 4-2.

Monocular Diplopia

If double vision persists even with one eye covered, then monocular diplopia is likely. Monocular diplopia is not caused by strabismus and, in the absence of an obvious cornea, pupil, or lens imperfection, is most typically refractive. Monocular diplopia caused by an uncorrected refractive error is typically described as an extra ghost image, often located vertically and very close to the original image. It disappears with a pinhole. It is corrected by a real refraction that

<table>
<tr><td colspan="4" align="center">Table 4-3
Exodeviations</td></tr>
<tr><td></td><td>**Fusion**</td><td>**Suppression**</td><td>**ARC?**</td></tr>
<tr><td>**Exophoria**</td><td>Yes</td><td>No</td><td>No</td></tr>
<tr><td>**Intermittent XT**</td><td>Yes</td><td>Yes</td><td>Maybe when tropic</td></tr>
<tr><td>**Exotropia**</td><td>No</td><td>Yes</td><td>Usually</td></tr>
</table>

searches for cylinder correction and uses the Jackson cross-cylinder, not just plus and minus over-correction. Monocular diplopia in both eyes can elicit two, three, or more images, all of which disappear with a pinhole.

Exodeviations

Exodeviations affect patients throughout their childhood and frequently into adulthood. While a patient may have been able to successfully remain asymptomatic as a child or young adult, adults with more stressful visual needs frequently succumb to the ever-present struggle to control their deviation comfortably. The result is generalized eye strain, horizontal diplopia, blurring, headache, fatigue with near work, or a debilitating combination of these.

The vast majority of exo patients are at some stage between being purely exophoric and being mostly exotropic. Many exo patients who go untreated start as phorias, then decompensate into intermittent tropias, and end up as constant exotropias (XTs). Throughout these changes, the size of the deviation does not vary much; most are between 20 to 30 prism diopters (PD). Most patients exhibit some degree of bicentral fusion and usually have equal or nearly equal vision.

Tropic time (the period during which the deviation is tropic) is most damaging to a young child because adaptations to strabismus occur most rapidly and easily at that age. Tropic time for adults frequently means diplopia and a sense of asthenopia and generates quizzical looks from others who wonder if their companion is looking at them. The clinician may get a false sense of the patient's control from measuring the patient only one time or at a particular time of day. Measuring fusional convergence amplitudes or observing fusional behavior with the cover–uncover test may also belie the patient's actual day-to-day control and comfort.

Careful history taking is more likely to reveal the ratio of straight versus tropic time if the adult patient knows when he or she is tropic. How much time a patient with an intermittent exotropia (X[T]) spends in the phoric state in comparison to how much time is spent in the tropic state must be noted. It is also necessary to determine if the XT is getting worse (decompensating) or staying the same. Be more specific than just asking, "Is the eye turn getting worse?" You must ask, "How many times daily does the eye deviate? When it does deviate, does it stay out for longer periods of time than previously?"

The symptoms of a decompensating adult exotrope will depend on his or her level of suppression and diplopia awareness when no longer fusing. Table 4-3 shows the different adaptive changes characteristic of exophorias, intermittent XTs, and constant XTs. Patients with an exophoria never suppress and always maintain bifoveal fusion, provided they have adequate convergence amplitudes. Remember that a phoria only manifests itself when fusion is disrupted,

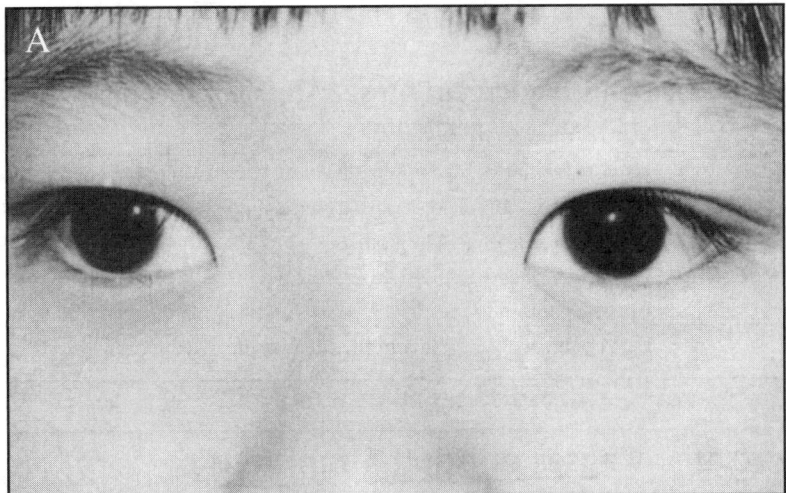

Figure 4-1. (A) Patient with large RXT (B) pulls straight and fuses with Polaroid glasses on for stereo testing.

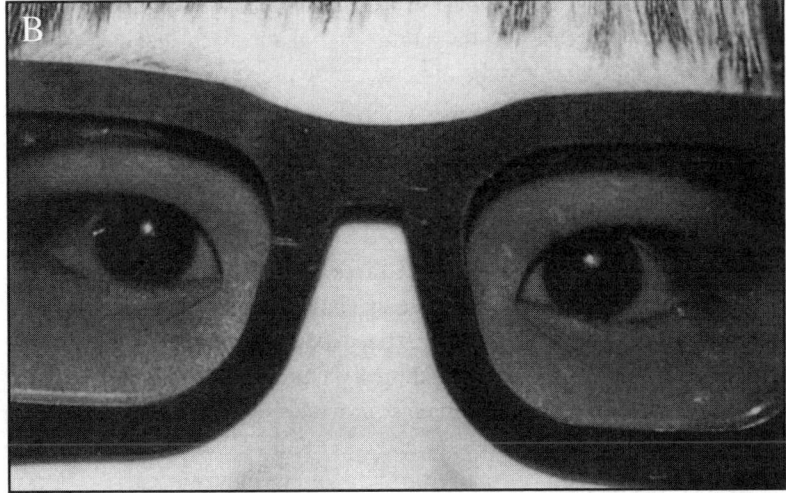

as with a cover–uncover test. With the eyes in the ortho position, the exophoric patient has NRC and good fusion.

Exophoric patients who suppress the temporal retina during bifoveal fixation will not appreciate diplopia if they slip into an exotropic position. One moment they could be straight and fixating bifoveally; the next moment they could be XT and suppressing with ARC. This is intermittent XT. Awareness of diplopia alerts an exotropic patient when the eyes start to slip into the tropic position. Teaching diplopia awareness may increase the control of patients with decompensating exodeviations, but only in patients who also have fusion potential.

Constant XTs are like X(T)s in their tropic state; they suppress and often have ARC. Although initially they might have been able to pull straight and fuse, once they have developed deep suppression, it is rare for them to ever pull straight. However, some patients who seem to have large, constant XTs actually can be briefly intermittent. These patients will pull straight during stereo testing once the Polaroid glasses are on (Figure 4-1). For the remainder of the exam—as with everyday seeing conditions—they have a constant XT, suppression, and no fusion.

Table 4-4
Systemic Diseases Causing Recent Onset Adult Strabismus

Disease	Strabismus Findings
Thyroid/Graves' disease	Usually restrictive, decreased elevation, often is initial symptom
Diabetes	CN III palsy (complete or partial) with pupil sparing, IV or VI
Myasthenia gravis	Any EOM palsy, including ptosis
Stroke/high blood pressure (HBP)	EOM palsy, hemianopic field defect
Arthritis	Brown syndrome
Tumor	EOM palsy with or without other neurological symptoms

Associated Causes of Adult Strabismus

Adult strabismus may be caused by a systemic illness. The astute clinician may, therefore, be the first step to diagnosing a systemic disease. While careful examination and diagnosis of the eye problem is the first step, the patient must also be directed to the proper medical care so that appropriate treatment can be initiated. The main systemic diseases that can cause recent onset strabismus in adults are listed in Table 4-4.

Graves' Disease—Thyroid Eye Disease

Patients with new diplopia and strabismus caused by Graves' disease may not be aware of their thyroid dysfunction. In fact, their thyroid blood tests may come out normal despite obvious involvement of the extraocular muscles (EOMs) by computerized axial tomography (CT) or magnetic resonance imaging (MRI) scanning, or simply their clinical picture. The patient with Graves' disease may also have one or all of the following problems: proptosis, lid retraction, decreased vision from optic nerve compression in a congested orbit, increased intraocular pressure, corneal problems from the inability to fully close the lids, and restriction of eye movements.

The strabismus exam for the patient with Graves' disease should include measurements in the nine diagnostic positions of gaze plus head tilt measurements (noting if the deviation is larger with either eye fixing). Because prism and cover (P + C) measurements require that the eyes move freely, your technique to measure patients with Graves' disease must be modified in this way. The correcting prism should be placed over the more restricted eye because it may be unable to fixate in the field of gaze that you are measuring. For instance, if the patient's right eye is restricted and is unable to elevate above the midline, upgaze measurements will be impossible with the right eye fixing. The right eye simply cannot fixate in upgaze. To measure by P + C then, place the correcting prism base up over the right eye and with the patient's chin down, have the more freely moving left eye fixate in upgaze. As you now cross-cover with the prism in place, the right eye will remain in its hypotropic position. If you have the correct amount of prism, neither eye will move. An astute patient will tell you that he or she is looking at the object of regard with the right eye only when you have the correct prism. He or she would not be able to actually "look at" the fixation target if you do not have the correct prism, even though he or she is trying to. If you have undercorrected the right hypo, the right eye of course will not move because it is restricted. The left eye, however, will respond with a slight downward motion to fixate, indicating that the deviation is undercorrected with the prism you have on the right eye.

This is not a DVD of the left eye but instead the restriction of the eye movements of the right eye causing the P + C measurements to be corrupted. If you have overcorrected the right hypo by using too much prism, the left eye will need to move slightly upward to fixate. In other words, since the right eye is never going to move in this situation because it is restricted, you are using the fixation movements of the left eye to guide your measurements. This technique is also used in extreme muscle palsies where the palsied eye also cannot move into the desired field of gaze for accurate P + C measurements.

Other measurements for the patient with Graves' disease are torsion measurement by double Maddox rods in the trial frame and versions and ductions (noting possible restrictions and lid lag from up to downgaze). Additionally, exophthalmometry measurements, intraocular pressure measured with the eye in primary position and again in attempted upgaze (looking for a rise in pressure in the upgaze measurement because of restricted globes), vision, and refraction should be done. Diplopia fields using a Goldmann-style perimeter may be useful. Stereopsis should be measured in the field of gaze in which the patient is able to see singly.

Finally, the examiner should try to identify if a correcting prism will alleviate the symptoms temporarily. Because the condition may be changing, a Fresnel press-on prism is initially preferred instead of an expensive ground-in prism. Prism correction is often marginally helpful due to the incomitant nature of the condition. Patients with the most success with prism tend to be those who appreciate that the area of single vision may be quite small and they need to move their head in order to keep the area straight ahead. Any torsional component may prevent any prism success. Occasionally, patients with Graves' disease will have convergence insufficiency, which may respond to standard convergence exercises. Some will actually have an EOM palsy. When strabismus surgery becomes necessary, it is performed after any decompression procedure but prior to any corrective lid surgery.

Muscle Palsy

EOM palsies may be caused by severe or subtle trauma. The patient may or may not have had loss of consciousness or may barely remember hitting his or her head after slipping on an icy sidewalk. Muscle palsies may also be caused by diabetes, myasthenia gravis, tumors, strokes, or frequently, no identifiable illness. They may resolve spontaneously, usually improving gradually within a few weeks of onset but taking as long as 1 year to disappear.

Stereopsis should be measured in the field of gaze where the patient is able to see singly. The examination should include measurements in the nine diagnostic positions of gaze plus head tilt measurements (noting if the deviation is larger with either eye fixing), torsion measurement by double Maddox rods in the trial frame, versions and ductions, plus vertical amplitudes for any vertical deviation, and horizontal (divergence and convergence) amplitudes for any horizontal deviation. These amplitude measurements, which are an assessment of the patient's motor fusion, are a critical measurement that will help determine if this is simply an old phenomenon that suddenly became noticeable or decompensated or if it is in fact a new phenomenon that requires further medical work-up. An old photograph may show that a compensatory head tilt existed previously. The Three Step Test, as described in Chapter 2, will help determine which muscle is palsied.

Diabetic Third Nerve Palsy

While diabetes can cause any of the EOM palsies, it classically causes the diabetic third nerve palsy. Its distinguishing feature from any other (congenital or acquired) third nerve palsy is that it spares the pupil. In other words, it has one or all of the features of a third nerve palsy (ptosis, eye down and out with medial rectus [MR], inferior rectus [IR], superior rectus [SR], inferior oblique [IO] weakness) but without the pupil being dilated. The pupils are absolutely normal.

The diabetic third nerve palsy usually resolves completely within a few weeks to a few months. Because of the distance between the diplopic images, the combined horizontal and vertical disparity, and the changeability of the diabetic third nerve palsy, prisms are not very useful. Occlusion may be used to eliminate diplopia. Patients with diabetes may develop cranial nerve (CN) IV (trochlear nerve) or CN VI (abducens nerve) palsies.

Myasthenia Gravis

New myasthenia gravis presents as diplopia 25% of the time. Its fatigability and variability give it away. One week the patient has a right fourth nerve palsy, the next week it might switch to the left. Prolonged attempted upgaze will typically cause either the eye to drop into a hypotropic position or the lid(s) to droop. Systemic treatment is required for the disease, but press-on prisms or occlusion may temporarily treat the ophthalmic findings. Strabismus surgery may be ultimately necessary once the disease stabilizes.

Progressive External Ophthalmoplegia

Progressive external ophthalmoplegia (PEO) is an insidious decrease in the ductional movements of the EOMs. Its progress is asymmetrical so that diplopia is often present in extreme gazes. While a specific muscle may not be identified as palsied, versions and ductions are limited. Patients find themselves moving their head more and more to get their eyes into a position in which they can see comfortably and singly.

Divergence Palsy

Divergence palsy, like the sixth nerve lateral rectus (LR) palsy, is a horizontal esodeviation that is classically worse at distance than at near. Unlike a sixth nerve palsy, however, the patient with divergence palsy has a horizontally comitant deviation and nonexistent base-in divergence amplitudes. It may be caused by encephalitis, multiple sclerosis, head trauma, or simply aging.

Blowout Fracture of the Orbit

Blunt trauma to the orbit may result in diplopia. While such diplopia may be caused simply by swelling with the orbit (restricting the eyes from moving properly), it may be caused by a fracture of the orbital bones and entrapment of one or more eye muscles. The strabismic work-up for such a patient should include measurements in the nine diagnostic positions of gaze, including head tilts, paying particular attention to the upgaze and downgaze measurements. Torsion should be noted by the double Maddox rods, and exophthalmometry measurements documenting proptosis or enophthalmos should be taken. Diplopia fields may be useful to document the remaining area of fusion. Stereopsis should be measured in the field of gaze that the patient is able to see singly.

Press-on prisms or occlusion may alleviate the patient's diplopia until it either resolves on its own or is surgically repaired by a team of ear, nose, and throat/orbital ophthalmic surgeons.

Convergence Insufficiency

One of the most likely causes of double vision in an adult is something frequently seen at all ages. Convergence insufficiency strikes at any age but is horribly debilitating to an older patient whose ability to read comfortably is extremely important. The patient may or may not have some form of exodeviation. Patients may complain of headaches after reading or doing near work, aching eyeballs, blurring (like a camera going in and out of focus), moving/swimming/jumping words, and losing their place (particularly at the end of a line). They may have true diplopia or admit to always closing one eye to read. Falling asleep after reading just a very short time is another common complaint.

Base-in prism should only be considered for the older patient who has failed at convergence exercises. Fortunately, exercises do work on these very desperate patients. Unfortunately, base-in prism is often prescribed as their first mode of treatment, and the certain demise of any convergence they might have is initiated. Base-in prism feels good at first and seems to cure their symptoms. However, because of the prism, they will exert less convergence. This will cause a further decrease in convergence, increased symptoms, and more dependence on their base-in prism glasses. Given these facts, patients rarely choose prism over exercises as a first treatment. Even very elderly patients will choose exercises at least as a first attempt to cure the problem.

Look for subtle differences in the baseline deviation, and remember that convergence is generally best in the downgaze reading position. If the patient complains that the newspaper is becoming difficult to read, try to determine exactly what is difficult. It may be that looking up to the top of the opened page is the real problem. In this case, the solution may be as simple as folding the paper and bringing it down to the normal reading position.

Decompensation Strabismus

Finally, older patients may present with a seemingly new problem that actually is a long-standing strabismus that just got worse. Small (or even large) esophorias, exophorias, and hypers may have been in control for years and the patient was completely asymptomatic. Suddenly, for no obvious reason (such as illness or trauma), the phoria may become less controlled and break down into an intermittent tropia. The patient may experience diplopia during the tropic phase and asthenopia while he or she is struggling to remain straight and single. All of this seems new. In the absence of an obvious cause, the most likely cause is simply a decompensated phoria. Treatment is aimed at relieving the symptoms.

Conclusion

When examining adults with strabismus, look beyond the eye problem and try to determine if there is a systemic problem causing the strabismus. Remember that the treatment is wholly dependent on the cause.

Resources

Grob D, Brunner NG, Namba T. The natural course of myasthenia gravis and effect of therapeutic measures. *Ann N Y Acad Sci.* 1981;377:652-669.

Hansen VC. Evaluation and management of monocular diplopia. *Am Orthoptic J.* 1994;44:50-55.

Hansen VC. *Ocular Motility.* Thorofare, NJ: SLACK Incorporated; 1988:87-88.

Harley RD. *Pediatric Ophthalmology.* Philadelphia, PA: WB Saunders; 1975:461.

Chapter 5

Extraocular Muscles— Anatomy and Function

KEY POINTS

- Understanding extraocular muscles (EOM) is essential in understanding EOM physiology and function.

- The cranial nerves that are responsible for ocular movements are III (oculomotor nerve), IV (trochlear nerve), and VI (abducens nerve).

- Duction is movement of one eye.

- Version is movement of both eyes in the same direction.

- The agonist muscle is the prime mover for a desired direction of gaze. The antagonist muscle of the same eye works directly against the agonist.

- Yoke muscles are pairs of muscles (one in each eye) that work together to achieve a desired version movement.

Eye Movements

The sophistication of our EOMs allows for many different kinds of eye movements. Moving the eye enables the field of view to increase and allows the fovea, the small region of best vision, to reposition itself as the object viewed changes. Our eyes can involuntarily follow a slow-moving object (smooth pursuit) or they can voluntarily jump from one object to another (saccade). Once we are viewing the new object, our eyes maintain fixation by constantly readjusting so that the object remains on the fovea (microsaccades). As our heads change position in space, information from the balancing apparatus in the inner ear sends messages to the EOMs to *right* the globes (vestibular). Our EOMs also use information from the position to sense mechanisms (proprioception). All of these eye movements can occur monocularly. Vergence movements allow both foveae to maintain fixation at the same time (bifoveal fixation) whether an object moves closer (and the eyes converge) or further away (and the eyes diverge). The rewards of maintaining bifoveal fixation are binocular vision and stereopsis.

So how do the individual EOMs work to accomplish all this? Say you are about to step off a curb. Suddenly, you stop and look to the left in time to see a taxi about to knock you off your feet. What did your visual system do? First, your brain received messages; you may have seen the moving taxi in the periphery of your retina, or you may have heard it, smelled it, or felt the wind from it. Perhaps you have learned about that particularly dangerous intersection. Something alerted your brain, which sent messages to the eye muscles telling them to move. (It also told your body to stop and tense up with adrenaline.) This occurred by nerve pathways.

Neurological Basis of Eye Movements

There are nerves from your brainstem, the part below the thinking cerebrum (which initiated your reaction), called the cranial nerves. The 12 cranial nerves are responsible for various duties both motor and sensory that help with basic functions (Table 5-1). The second cranial nerve (CN II) is the sensory nerve responsible for vision, but it is three other cranial nerves (CNs III, IV, and VI) that are involved in ocular movement. This anatomy in the brain is important because it sets the scene for many EOM syndromes and locates neurological diseases that affect the eye muscles in specific but unusual ways.

Bony Orbit

The globe is located in a part of the skull known as the orbit. The orbit includes portions of seven bones—maxilla, frontal, zygomatic, sphenoid, palatine, ethmoid, and lacrimal. This bony orbit provides protection for the eyeball as well as an anchor for the EOMs.

The lateral and medial walls of each orbit form a 45-degree angle with each other, and the medial walls of each eye are parallel to each other so that the lateral walls of each eye form a 90-degree angle to each other. The two openings in the back of the orbit, the orbit's apex, are the optic foramen and the superior orbital fissure. The rounder, more nasal, and slightly inferior optic foramen allows passage of the optic nerve and central retinal artery from the brain to the globe. The elongated superior orbital fissure allows passage of the nerves to the EOMs and globe and the venous flow from the orbit.

Table 5-1
Nature and Function of Cranial Nerves

Cranial Nerves	Sensory/Motor	Function
I. Olfactory	Sensory	Smell
II. Optic	Sensory	Vision
III. Oculomotor	Motor	Levator, pupil constriction, SR, MR, IR, IO
IV. Troclear	Motor	SO
V. Trigeminal: Ophthalmic Maxillary Mandibular	Both	Lacrimal, frontal, nasociliary
VI. Abducens	Motor	LR
VII. Facial	Both	Facial expression Facial sensation
VIII. Vestibulocochlear	Sensory	Hearing, equilibrium
IX. Glossopharyngeal	Both	Taste, salivation, motor to pharynx
X. Vagus	Both	Visceral sensory, motor to pharynx, and larynx
XI. Accessory	Motor	Larynx, sternocleidomastoid, and trapezius
XII. Hypoglossal	Motor	Tongue

Extraocular Muscles

The annulus of Zinn is a ring of connective tissue attached to the inside of the orbital apex. The EOMs, except the inferior oblique (IO), attach and originate the annulus of Zinn and course forward through orbital tissue to attach to the globe. Each muscle becomes tendon that attaches to the globe. The length of the tendon varies from one muscle to another, as does the location of attachment. The muscles are composed of different types of tissue, allowing for quick bursts of activity (saccades) as well as slow, precise movements (pursuit). The muscle fibers are in constant state of readiness, or tonus.

When the head is erect, the eye assumes the primary position in the orbit with the fovea pointed straight ahead at the horizon. The visual axis is the imaginary line between the fovea and the object of regard.

The muscle plane includes the center of rotation of the globe, the particular muscle's insertion on the globe, and the muscle's origin. The muscle contracts back toward its firmly fixed origin, pulling the globe around its center of rotation, from the muscle's insertion.

Imagine a yo-yo on its side as you pull the string backward. The front of the yo-yo (the corneal apex) will rotate around its center toward the finger pulling the string (the origin). Now tilt the yo-yo halfway up on its side. As you pull back, the front of the yo-yo moves back (but less efficiently) and up. So even though you are pulling the same string, there is a different action. In the same way, the individual muscle action changes when the eye moves and the visual axis and muscle plane no longer coincide.

This explains why the medial rectus (MR) and lateral rectus (LR) have only one action—their muscle planes naturally coincide with the eye's visual axis (Figure 5-1). The muscle planes of the other EOMs (superior rectus [SR], inferior rectus [IR], superior oblique [SO], and inferior

Figure 5-1. Relationship of visual axis to the muscle place of MR.

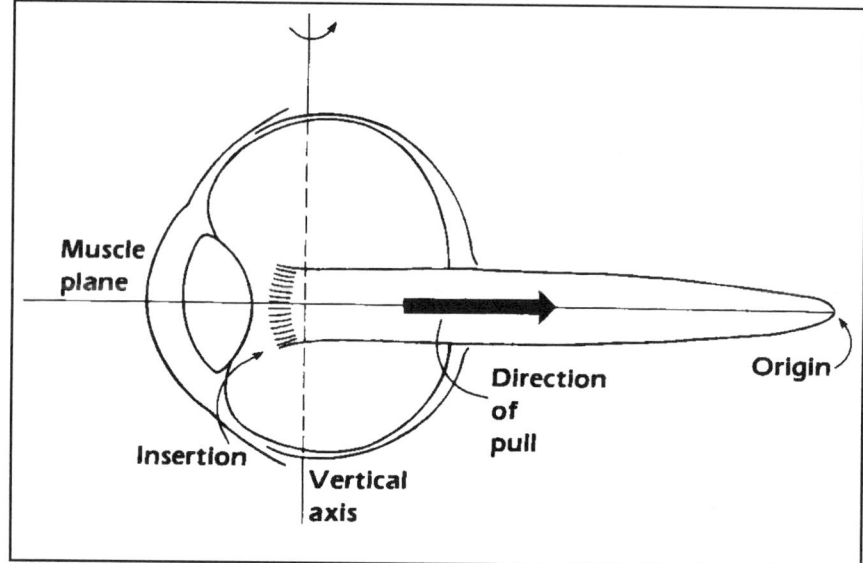

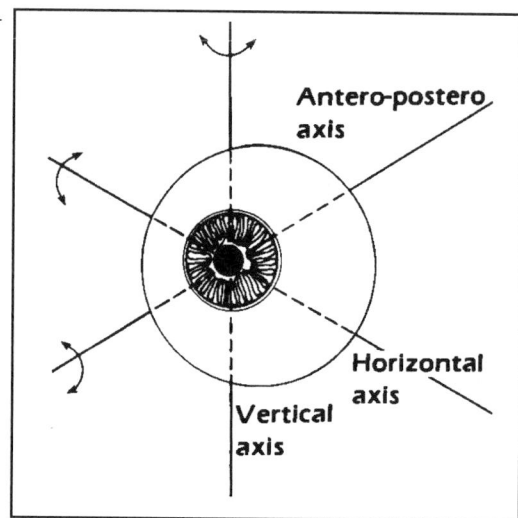

Figure 5-2. Axes of the globe—horizontal, vertical, and antero-postero.

oblique [IO]) do *not* naturally coincide with the visual axis when the eye is in the primary position. When those cyclovertical muscles contract, the movement is a combination of vertical action (around the horizontal axis), horizontal action (around the vertical axis), and the torsional action (around the antero–postero axis) (Figure 5-2). Remember that a muscle does not *push* the eye around; it contracts back toward its fixed origin, pulling the eye with it from its insertion on the globe.

The cyclovertical muscles have three actions. The primary action of a muscle is the main action occurring when the eye is in the primary position. This primary action increases when the eye moves from primary position into ABDuction. The secondary action of a muscle has less influence but increases when the eye moves into ADDuction. The tertiary action is minor but is either ADDuction or ABDuction.

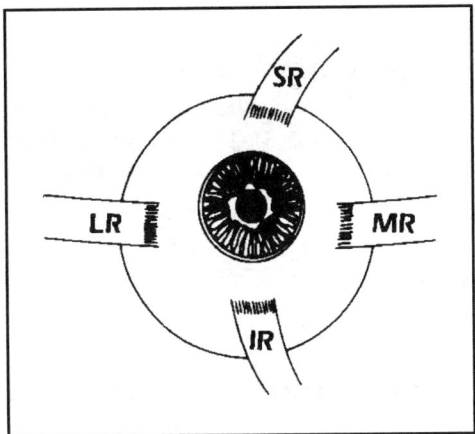

Figure 5-3. Position of insertions of the four rectus muscles, right eye.

Medial Rectus

The MR inserts 5.5 mm behind the limbus on the medial side of the globe (Figure 5-3). This muscle is an average of 41 mm long with 4 mm of tendon. The average width of the tendinous insertion on the globe is 10.5 mm. The MR is innervated by the inferior division of the oculomotor nerve (CN III), and the muscle originates at the annulus of Zinn. Its function is to rotate the eye medially toward the nose; it ADDucts the eye. With the eye in primary position, the MR muscle plane coincides perfectly with the eye's visual axis. The MR is slightly more effective in downgaze, the reading position, and when the eye fixates at near positions.

The MR is the strongest EOM for two reasons. First, its insertion is more anterior on the globe than the other muscles, and therefore, it has a significant wrap-around effect. Second, the MR weighs the most. Humans use the MR a lot (for reading), which probably accounts for its advanced development.

Lateral Rectus

The LR also works horizontally about the vertical axis, but because it inserts on the globe on the lateral (temporal) side (see Figure 5-3), it rotates the eye temporally; it ABDucts the eye. It inserts 7 mm behind the limbus, and the average width of its insertion is 9.5 mm. The LR originates at the annulus of Zinn. Its average length is 40.5 mm, with 8.5 mm of tendon. It is the only EOM that is innervated by the abducens nerve (CN VI). The LR is also the only rectus muscle that is supplied by only one anterior ciliary artery, although new studies suggest this is not true. (The other three rectus muscles have two each; the oblique muscles have none.) The LR muscle plane coincides perfectly with the visual axis when the eye is in the primary position and, therefore, its only action is ABDuction. The LR works most effectively during distance fixation and upgaze (in contrast to the MR).

Cyclovertical Muscles

The muscle planes of the remaining four cyclovertical muscles do not coincide with the visual axis and, therefore, each muscle has horizontal, vertical, and torsional capabilities. Although the muscle plane cannot change much, the visual axis can. Thus, depending on where the eye looks, these actions change. In some positions, the muscle plane and visual axis will be closer to lining up than in other positions.

Superior Rectus

The SR originates at the annulus of Zinn and travels forward above the globe and SO muscle but underneath the levator lid muscle. It inserts 7.7 mm behind the limbus on the superior side of the globe, farther back than any other rectus muscle (see Figure 5-3). The average length of the SR is 42 mm. The average length of its tendon is 5.5 mm, and its tendon width is 10.5 mm. Innervation to the SR is by the superior division of the oculomotor nerve (CN III).

When the eye is in the primary position, the SR muscle plane forms an angle of 23 degrees with the eye's visual axis (Figure 5-4). When the eye ABDucts exactly 23 degrees, the visual axis coincides exactly with the SR muscle plane. At this position, when the SR contracts, the eye goes straight up. The function of the SR is pure elevation when the eye is ABDucted 23 degrees. The SR *alone* may be tested when the patient is instructed to elevate the eye from the ABDucted position. Elevation is the primary action of the SR, and like all cyclovertical actions, this primary action increases in ABDuction and decreases in ADDuction.

When the eye rotates exactly 67 degrees into ADDuction, the visual axis moves to make a 90-degree angle with the SR muscle plane. When the SR contracts at this position, it has no effect on elevation but rotates the globe about the antero–postero axis. This intorts the eye so that the 12 o'clock position of the cornea rotates nasally. Intorsion is the secondary action of the SR.

The insertion of the SR on the globe is anterior to the equator (the imaginary ring that cuts the eye in half front to back) and relatively temporal to its origin at the annulus of Zinn. Thus, when the SR contracts, it pulls the front of the eyes nasally and slightly ADDucts the eye. ADDuction is the tertiary action of the SR.

Inferior Rectus

Like the SR, the IR originates at the annulus of Zinn and travels downward, then forward beneath the globe, and inserts relatively temporal to its origin, 6.5 mm behind the limbus (see Figure 5-3). Its average length is 40 mm, its tendon 5 mm, and it width 10 mm at the insertion. The IR is innervated by the inferior division of the oculomotor nerve (CN III). The IR works closely with the IO, the lower lid eye muscles, and the ligament of Lockwood (the hammock-like structure that helps support the globe). For this reason, complications involving the lower lid can arise following excessive surgery on the IR.

The muscle plane on the IR forms an angle 23 degrees with the visual axis when the eye is in the primary position (as with the SR) (see Figure 5-4). When the eye ABDucts exactly 23 degrees, the IR muscle plane coincides perfectly with the visual axis. If the eye looks down from that 23 degrees ABDucted position, the depression is due to the IR alone. The primary action of the IR is depression. This action increases in ABDuction and decreases to nonexistence in ADDuction. To see if the IR is working properly, direct the patient to look 23 degrees into ABDuction and then look down. If the eye moves down from that ABDucted position, the IR is working properly.

When the eye ADDucts exactly 67 degrees and the IR contracts, no vertical movement is being generated because the new visual axis position now forms a 90-degree angle with the IR muscle plane. The only action from ADDuction is movement about the antero–postero axis. When the IR contracts, the eye will extort so that the 12 o'clock position of the cornea rotates temporally. Extorsion is the secondary action of the IR.

Like the SR, the IR insertion on the globe is anterior to the equator and relatively temporal to its origin. Thus, when the IR contracts, it has a slight ADDucting effect. The tertiary action of

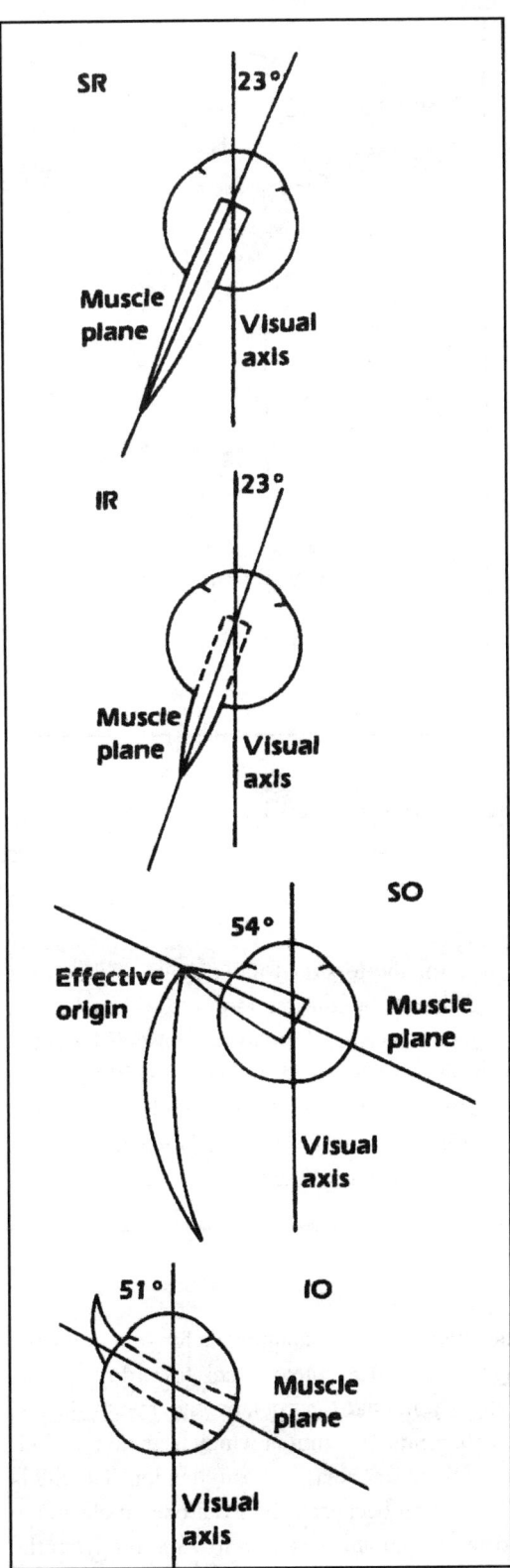

Figure 5-4. The four cyclovertical muscles, illustrating the angle between the muscle plane and visual axis with the eyes in the primary position.

Figure 5-5. Relationship between SO and SR of the right eye.

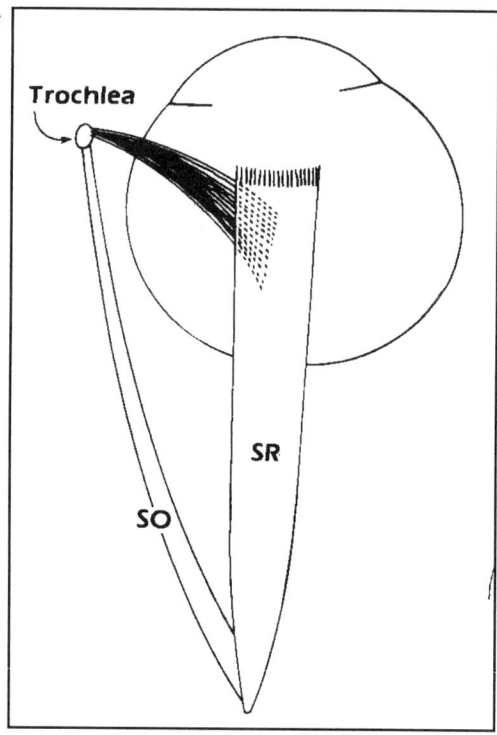

the IR is ADDuction. So the SR and IR work together as ADDuctors but against each other as torters and vertically acting muscles.

Oblique Muscles

The two oblique muscles are mainly responsible for the torsional movements of the globe and for maintaining a forward pulling force on the globe. If the four recti muscles relaxed as the two oblique muscles contracted, the eye literally pops forward. The oblique muscles keep the eye in the upright 12 o'clock position, despite the position of the head (ie, when the head tilts to the right shoulder, both eyes rotate to the left shoulder; the right eye intorts, the left eye extorts). The muscle planes of both oblique muscles do not coincide with the visual axis when the eye is in the primary position. These cyclovertical muscles also have three actions that vary depending on the eye's position.

Superior Oblique

The SO originates at the back of the orbit at the annulus of Zinn and travels forward along the medial–superior side of the orbit. It passes through the trochlea, reflects back toward the globe, fans out, and inserts onto the top of the globe slightly behind the equator underneath the SR (Figure 5-5). The average length of the entire SO is 59.5 mm, 19.5 mm of which is tendon. In fact, the reflected part of the muscle (after it passes through the trochlea) is mostly tendon. The SO is the eye's longest muscle. Its width varies from 7 to 18 mm because it fans out once it clears the trochlea. The muscle insertion runs anterior to posterior and attaches 13.8 to 18.8 mm from the limbus. The SO is innervated solely by the trochlear nerve (CN IV).

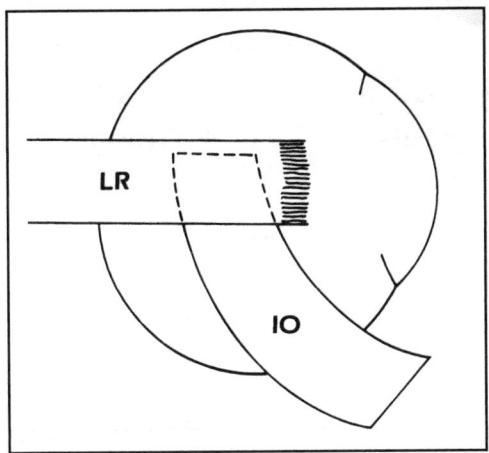

Figure 5-6. Relationship between the IO and LR of the right eye.

Despite its origin at the annulus of Zinn, the SO's effective origin is at the trochlea. When the SO contracts, it pulls the top of the globe forward and toward the trochlea. Mechanical limitations in and around the trochlea can limit the effectiveness of the SO. For this reason, the SO is extremely susceptible to mild trauma or inflammation around the trochlea.

The muscle plane of the SO is formed by its reflected portion and includes the trochlea and the insertion of the SO on the globe. Thus the muscle plane is at a 54-degree angle to the visual axis when the eye is in primary position (see Figure 5-4). The primary action of the SO is intorsion. When the eye ABDucts exactly 36 degrees, the visual axis forms at a 90-degree angle with the SO muscle plane. When the SO contracts from this position, it intorts the globe around the antero–postero axis.

With the globe ADDucted exactly 54 degrees, the visual axis and muscle plane precisely coincide. When the SO contracts in this position, it acts as a pure depressor, pulling the top of the globe forward toward the trochlea. Thus, the secondary action of the SO is depression even though the muscle attaches superiorly on the globe. With the eye in ADDuction, the primary action (intorsion) of the SO decreases.

Because the SO inserts slightly behind the equator and the effective origin (trochlea) is relatively medial to its insertion on the globe, the SO pulls the *back* of the eye nasally (toward the trochlea) when it contracts. This results in the *front* of the eye ABDucting about the vertical axis. Thus the tertiary action of the SO is ABDuction.

Inferior Oblique

The IO is the only EOM whose true origin is not the annulus of Zinn. The IO originates at the posterior lacrimal crest of the infero–nasal orbital rim margin. The muscle travels back in the orbit, underneath the globe and IR (but within Lockwood's ligament), and curves up underneath the LR. Its posterior edge inserts 1 mm anterior to and below the fovea. The anterior edge inserts approximately 17 mm behind the limbus (Figure 5-6). It is innervated by the inferior division of the oculomotor nerve (CN III).

The muscle plane of the IO forms a 51-degree angle with the visual axis when the eye is in primary position (see Figure 5-4). When the IO contracts, it pulls from its insertion toward its origin (the inferior nasal orbital rim). This extorts the eye. Extorsion is the primary action of the IO. If the eye is ABDucted exactly 39 degrees, the IO muscle plane forms a 90-degree angle with

Table 5-2
Muscle Information

Muscle	Length	Limbus to Insertion	Muscle Plane Angle
MR	41 mm	5.5 mm	0 degrees
LR	40.5 mm	7.0 mm	0 degrees
SR	42 mm	7.7 mm	23 degrees
IR	40 mm	6.5 mm	23 degrees
SO	59.5 mm*	13.8 to 18.8 mm	54 degrees
IO	37 mm	17 mm	51 degrees

*SO total length, 19.5 mm of it is tendon

Table 5-3
Muscle Actions and Testing Positions

Muscle	Actions: 1°/2°/3°	Test
MR	Only ADDucts	ADDuction
LR	Only ABDucts	ABDuction
SR	Elevation/intorsion/ADDuction	Out/up
IR	Depression/extorsion/ADDuction	Out/down
SO	Intorsion/depression/ABDuction	In/down
IO	Extorsion/elevation/ABDuction	In/up

the visual axis. Contraction of the muscle will then result in pure extorsion of the globe around the antero–postero axis.

Again, the primary action decreases in ADDuction. With the globe ADDucted exactly 51 degrees, the IO muscle plane coincides with the visual axis. Contraction of the IO in this position results in the secondary action of elevation (even though the IO is inferior to the globe).

The IO inserts behind the equator and temporal to its origin. When it contracts, the IO pulls the back of the globe medially so that the front of the eye ABDucts. Thus, the tertiary action of the IO is ABDuction.

Summary of Muscle Actions

Table 5-2 outlines important information about each EOM. Table 5-3 shows the actions and testing positions for each EOM. As previously stated, to test the SR you instruct the patient to ABDuct 23 degrees and then elevate the globe. Although the SR itself is an ADDuctor, its function is tested in the out and up position. While the SR and IR can be tested by asking the patient to perform the primary action of each (elevation and depression, respectively), the SO and IO cannot be tested in this way. You cannot ask the patient to intort the eye using the SO! You can, however, ask the patient to show the vertical action of the SO and IO. To do this, you first have the patient take the eye into ADDuction, then elevate (IO function) or depress (SO function).

	Table 5-4	
	Synergists/Antagonists	
Muscle	**Synergists**	**Antagonists**
MR	SR, IR	LR, SO, IO
LR	SO, IO	MR, SR, IR
SR	Elevation: IO	IR, SO
	Intorsion: SO	IR, IO
	ADDuction: MR, IR	LR, SO, IO
IR	Depression: SO	SR, IO
	Extorsion: IO	SR, SO
	ADDuction: MR, SR	LR, SO, IO
SO	Intorsion: SR	IO, IR
	Depression: IR	SR, IO
	ABDuction: LR, IO	MR, SR, IR
IO	Extorsion: IR	SO, SR
	Elevation: SR	IR, SO
	ABDuction: LR, SO	MR, SR, IR

The mnemonic "SIN RAD" will help you remember the torsional and horizontal actions of the cyclovertical muscles. "SIN" means that the Superior muscles INtort; so conversely, the two inferior muscles must extort. "RAD" means that the Recti muscles ADDuct; so the obliques must ABDuct.

Descriptive Muscle Terms

The agonist muscle is the prime mover for a desired direction of gaze. The antagonist muscle of the same eye works directly against the agonist. The MR is the agonist for ADDuction; the LR is its direct antagonist. A muscle in the same eye that helps another muscle accomplish a particular action is called a synergist muscle. So both the SO and IO are synergists for ABDuction with the LR. But these same two muscles, the SO and IO, are antagonists for torsional and vertical action. Table 5-4 shows the synergist–antagonist relationship among the six EOMs for horizontal, vertical, and torsional actions.

Yoke muscles are pairs of muscles (one in each eye) that work together to achieve a desired version movement (Figures 5-7 and 5-8). Duction is movement of one eye. Version is movement of both eyes in the same direction. Dextroversion is movement of both eyes to the right; levoversion is movement of both eyes to the left. The terms *supraversion* for upgaze and *infraversion* for downgaze are seldom used.

Laws Governing Eye Movements

Two basic laws govern how innervation is supplied to an agonist, its antagonist, and yoke. Sherrington's law of reciprocal innervation applies to the agonist and antagonist of one eye. Every unit of innervation to the agonist is accompanied by a reciprocal amount of relaxation to

Figure 5-7. Pairs of yoke muscles responsible for moving eyes into various positions of gaze.

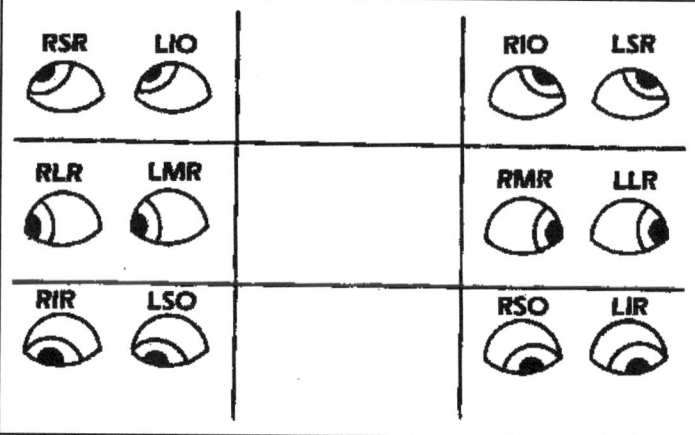

Figure 5-8. Schematic drawing of muscles responsible for moving eyes into tertiary positions.

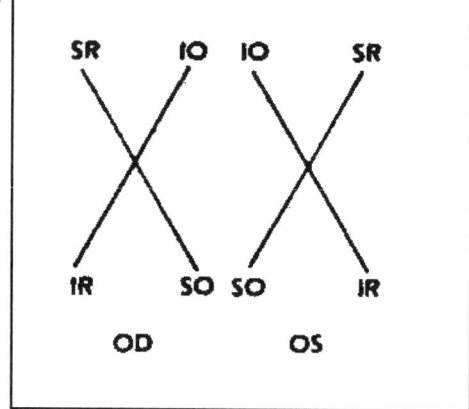

the antagonist muscle. For example, as the MR contracts a given amount, its antagonist—the LR—relaxes an equal reciprocal amount.

Hering's law of simultaneous innervation applies to the yoke muscles of each eye. The fixing, or "driving," eye determines how much innervation goes to the agonist of that eye; an equal amount of innervation then goes to its yoke in the other eye. When all of the muscles are healthy and working at normal levels, the eyes remain parallel, regardless of where they turn together.

When one muscle is weak, or palsied, the system is no longer perfectly balanced. For example, if the right MR (RMR) was palsied, more innervation than usual would be required to move that eye into ADDuction. Its direct antagonist, the right LR (RLR), would then require less innervation to move the eye into ABDuction because it would be pulling against a weak muscle. The yoke muscles of the RMR and RLR would also be affected because they would receive equal, but inappropriate, innervation. If the palsied right eye was fixing and moving into the field of action of the palsied RMR, its yoke (the left LR [LLR]) would receive the same amount of extra innervation and would overshoot into ABDuction. In dextroversion, the RLR's yoke (the left MR [LMR]) would receive the same amount of innervation and would appear underactive because its own direct antagonist is a healthy LLR.

Version testing assesses how well a pair of yoke muscles work together based on Hering's law. For example, when looking up and to the left, the right IO and left SR should pull both eyes up together to the desired position of gaze. Each eye should have moved with equal speed and smoothness and should be at the same height with respect to each other. This would be a normal version movement.

If one eye becomes the fixing eye and the other slows down and never achieves the same position as the fixing eye, an underactive muscle is indicated. Ductions of the eye with the apparent underaction should be performed. If the weakness is still apparent, there is either a restriction holding back the eye or possibly a severe muscle palsy. If, instead, the nonfixing eye had sped up and passed the desired position during version testing, the muscle is considered overactive. You must then determine if it is a primary overaction or a secondary overaction. A secondary overaction is due to an underactive antagonist. A primary overaction occurs without an antagonist underaction; it simply occurs.

Resources

Duane TD, ed. *Clinical Ophthalmology.* Vol. 1. Harper & Row.

Frank J. *Oculomotor Physiology* [section of Orthoptic Basic Science Videotape Series]. Madison, WI: American Orthoptic Council.

Havertape S. *Ocular Anatomy* [section of Orthoptic Basic Science Videotape Series]. Madison, WI: American Orthoptic Council.

Nemeth SC, Shea CA. *Medical Sciences for the Ophthalmic Assistant.* Thorofare, NJ: SLACK Incorporated; 1988.

Parks M. *Ocular Anatomy and Strabismus.* New York, NY: Harper & Row; 1975.

Von Noorden GK. *Binocular Vision and Ocular Motility.* Philadelphia, PA: Mosby; 1996.

Chapter 6

Binocularity

- Stereoscopic three-dimensional vision is the result of fusing the slightly different images that each eye sees when viewing an object binocularly.

- Good motor fusion implies that the patient has good sensory fusion.

- Abnormal binocularity is the brain's attempt to cope with strabismus.

Binocularity Defined

Humans and a few other animal species have binocularity. That is, we have the advantage of being able to use both eyes together in order to achieve an advanced level of vision. Simply put, we are able to appreciate seeing our world in depth—in a three-dimensional way. Having two eyes is more than just nature's safeguard in case one eye is blinded. It affords us a unique dimension to our visual skills. Yet people who have never had binocularity do not miss it, just as a person with color deficiency never complains that his grass really is not greener, or a child with 20/200 vision from ocular albinism rarely complains of poor vision. Patients without true binocularity since birth do not really know what they are missing.

Binocularity is a broad term that refers to the use of the two eyes together, either correctly (normally) or incorrectly (abnormally or anomalously). Normal binocularity often results in comfortable three-dimensional vision, or stereopsis. True stereopsis is the three-dimensional vision that you can have only with normal binocularity and normal vision. Fusion, then, is a type of binocularity in which the blending of two images, one from each eye, creates a single image in the brain. Stereopsis occurs because each eye sees a slightly different view of the object due to the position of the eyes in your head. Try focusing on one object and then comparing the view of the right eye to the left eye. The difference is subtle because of the spacing of the eyes in the skull, but it is still fusible because each eye's view so closely overlaps the other.

The ability to judge depth does exist without stereopsis, however. Visual clues such as overlap of contours or the apparent converging of parallel lines give a person a sense of depth without true stereopsis. Thus, a patient with one eye can be aware of depth perception but not have true stereopsis.

Fusion

There are two types of fusion: sensory and motor. Sensory fusion occurs in your brain. Motor fusion is the coordinated eye movements that are performed in order to maintain sensory fusion. A simple example of this is the alignment adjustment you would make while watching a car move closer to you. As it moves toward you, your eyes must converge. If your eyes do not have motor fusion to converge on the car (keeping the image of the car on each fovea), sensory fusion of the car will stop, and double vision will result. The existence of good motor fusion generally means that there is good sensory fusion.

The converse is not true—excellent sensory fusion does not automatically mean excellent (or even adequate) motor fusion. An example of this is the patient with immobile eye muscles due to Graves' thyroid ophthalmopathy. With the compensatory head position, the person might have bifoveal stereoscopic sensory fusion but will not have amplitudes of motor fusion.

Table 6-1 lists tests for sensory fusion (some of which are also stereo tests). Table 6-2 lists tests for stereoacuity. Table 6-3 lists tests used exclusively for evaluating motor fusion.

Normal Versus Abnormal Binocularity

Normal binocularity is the result of straight eyes and the brain's recognition of that fact. Persons with binocularity appreciate stereopsis when the conditions are right and see double (diplopia) when those conditions change.

Table 6-1

Tests for Sensory Fusion

- Stereo tests
- Worth four-dot
- Haploscopic devices (synoptophore, troposcope, amblyoscope)
- Red filter
- Bagolini lenses

Table 6-2

Tests for Stereoacuity

- Titmus
- Randot tests
- Lang
- Frisby
- Haploscopic devices

Table 6-3

Exclusive Motor Fusion Tests

- Vergence amplitudes (convergence, divergence, vertical, or torsional)
- 4-diopter base-out

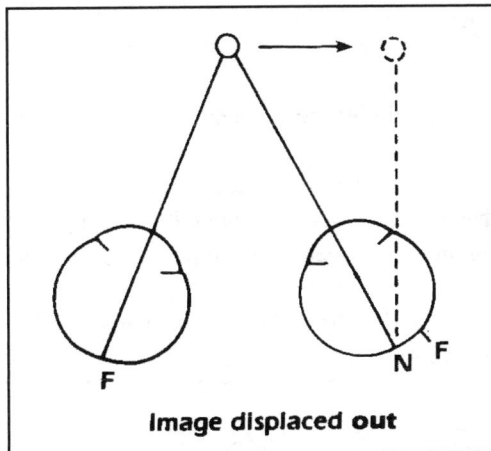

Image displaced out

Figure 6-1. Eye IN, extra image OUT.

Diplopia results when the image of a single object falls on the fovea of one eye and on a non-foveal point of the deviated second eye. Monocular projection determines that the right half of the retina is responsible for seeing objects located in the left half of the field. Therefore, binocular diplopia results in the image from the deviated eye being perceived as oppositely located. An eye that is crossed IN perceives the "extra" image to have moved OUT (Figure 6-1). This simple explanation helps interpret the results of the so-called diplopia tests. Whether using the red glass test for diplopia, the Maddox rod test for measuring strabismus, or Worth four-dot test for fusion, the patient's response is always the same in the case of normal binocularity with straight eyes:

fusion, or the blending of the two images. The response changes to diplopia when strabismus occurs in patients with normal binocularity. If the eye is crossed IN, the extra image, red light, red Maddox rod line, or red lights of the Worth four-dot are always perceived as having moved OUTward so that the crossed eye sees the image on the same side. Likewise, an eye that is deviated UP produces an extra image that is displaced DOWNward.

Abnormal binocularity is the brain's attempt to cope with a tropia in a visually immature patient. This may result in either rudimentary fusion or suppression in an attempt to get rid of the extra image.

Abnormal retinal correspondence is the brain's attempt to fuse in spite of eyes that are not straight. In the younger, visually immature patient, it is an adaptation by the brain to make the best of the deviated eye. In abnormal retinal correspondence, patients will subjectively tell you that they perceive fusion when, objectively, you have determined a frank tropia.

In older, visually mature tropic patients, the significance of ARC is most important when considering corrective strabismus surgery. A new problem (diplopia) will surface if the brain does not like its new postoperative eye position. While many patients will experience diplopia in the immediate postoperative period, the majority will not be bothered by permanent diplopia. It is therefore helpful to try to predict which patients will be likely to have persistent diplopia postoperatively. The best preoperative test in this case is to artificially put the eyes into their new position with prisms. Some patients immediately adapt to the new position and will tolerate strabismus surgery without permanent postoperative diplopia. Other patients will need a little more practice and may benefit from wearing the corrective prism for a longer period of time. Fresnel press-on prisms are designed for wear on a patient's existing glasses and are ideal in this situation. If the patient does not wear glasses, your local optical shop can arrange for the patient to borrow a loaner frame with plano lenses.[1]

The second type of abnormal binocularity is suppression, in which the brain "shuts off" the deviated eye. When both eyes are open, the image from the deviated eye is not perceived. If that eye is forced into use by covering the fixing eye, the vision will be normal. However, if both eyes are again allowed to look, the brain will selectively shut off the deviated eye. This is called suppression.

In more extreme cases, forcing the suppressed eye to look by covering the fixing eye still does not allow the eye to see normally. Poor vision in that eye persists, even though it is the only eye trying to see. Corrective eyeglass lenses will not improve the vision. This type of suppression, which persists under monocular conditions, is a form of amblyopia.

Detection of fusion, motor and sensory, and assessment of the patient's binocular status is a critical part of the ophthalmic work-up of a patient with strabismus.

Reference

1. Hansen VC, Freeman RS, Swarbrick CB. *Long Versus Short Term Prism Adaptation in Adults.* Stockholm, Sweden: Transactions IX International Orthoptic Congress; 1999.

Chapter 7

Differential Diagnosis— Ins, Outs, Ups, and Downs

KEY POINTS

- Initial information gathered by history taking and the basic work-up provides the clinician with a list of potential diagnoses or a differential diagnosis.

- The differential diagnosis is narrowed down by performing additional tests that eliminate or confirm each potential diagnosis.

Using the Differential Diagnosis

The mechanics of completing a motility exam are only half of your examination. The second half is putting all the information together to come up with a working diagnosis. To get there takes more than simply walking through the four-part exam of history, fusion, alignment, and vision. Additional tests must be added when necessary and interpreted accurately in order to put the pieces together into a working diagnosis. Once you have arrived at the diagnosis, the treatment plan can be formulated and carried out.

A working differential diagnosis begins with a thought process that leads an examiner through the exam to a final diagnosis. The patient's history, appearance, and age provide the first clues. A final diagnosis is reached through the process of elimination and on the basis of test results but only if the examiner performed the appropriate tests in the proper sequence to avoid examination pollution.

The following tables (Tables 7-1 through 7-14) address the different types of strabismus by listing a tentative diagnosis, the additional history that will be helpful to secure the diagnosis, along with the appropriate tests (and their results) that will clinch the diagnosis.

Table 7-1

Esodeviations

Tentative Diagnosis

1. **Infantile ET**

   a. *Additional history:*

   Onset before age 6 months

   Fixates with either eye

   Constant ET

   b. *Test:*   *Indicates:*

   ABDuction   Reluctant but intact

   Measurements   Large ET, V pattern often

   Cross-fixates   Equal vision

   Cycloplegic refraction   Small refractive error

   Versions   Possible IO overaction

   Cover-uncover   Possible DVD

2. **Accommodative ET**

   a. *Additional history:*

   E(T), N>D

   Eye preference

   Worse when tired, concentrating

   Typical age of onset 18 months to 3 years

   Range of onset 7 months to 10 years

   b. *Test:*   *Indicates:*

   P + C, cc + sc   Accommodative component

   Cycloplegic refraction   <4 D hyperopia, usually high AC/A

                                                  >4 D hyperopia, usually normal AC/A

   Fusion, cc   Usually excellent

   Vision   Frequent amblyopia

3. **LR palsy (CN VI)**

   a. *Additional history:*

   Severe head/neck trauma

   ET greater to right gaze, left gaze, or both sides

   Head position to right or left

   Variable horizontal diplopia, worse at distance

   Sudden onset of ET/diplopia

   Present since birth if congenital

   Associated with facial nerve palsy

      (Moebius or brainstem tumor)

   Associated with ear pain (Gradenigo)

   Worsens with fatigue (myasthenia gravis)

(continued)

Table 7-1 (continued)

Esodeviations

3. **LR palsy (CN VI) (continued)**

   b. *Test:*   *Indicates:*

   Fusion using head position   Recent onset
   Measurements   ET> right and/or left gaze
                                           ET D>N, slight A tendency
   Measure with OD, OS fix   Primary/secondary deviation
   Versions/ductions, saccades   Decreased LR function
   Diplopia testing   Horizontal, incomitant
                                           Young child may suppress
   Vision   Possible amblyopia if early onset
   Forced ductions   Negative unless very longstanding with
                                              resultant MR contracture

4. **Duane retraction syndrome, type 1**

   a. *Additional history:*
   No trauma
   Lid fissure changes with gaze
   Abnormal head position
   Present since birth

   b. *Test:*   *Indicates:*
   Versions, ductions   No ABDuction, lid fissure narrows during
                                              ADDuction
   Fusion with head position   Frequently fuses
   Vision   Possible amblyopia

5. **Consecutive ET**

   a. *Additional history:*
   Previous surgery for XT

   b. *Test*   *Indicates:*
   Fusion with ET corrected   Usually fuses if X or X(T) preop

6. **Nystagmus compensation syndrome**

   a. *Additional history:*
   Nystagmus during ABDuction
   Large ET present since birth
   Cross-fixates, turns head to see

   b. *Test:*   *Indicates:*
   Krimsky   Overconverges with correcting prism
   Versions/ductions   Jerk nystagmus in ABDuction, both eyes
   Cross-fixation   Does not move fixing eye out of
                                              ADDucted position to mid-line

(continued)

Table 7-1 (continued)

Esodeviations

7. **Cyclic ET**
    a. *Additional history:*
        24-, 48-, or 96-hour schedule of alternation
            between ET one cycle and straight next cycle
        Fairly sudden onset during childhood

    b. *Test:*   *Indicates:*

ET day:	Fusion	Initially may have diplopia, then suppression/ARC
	P + C	Large ET, usually comitant
	Vision	May have amblyopia eventually
Straight day:	Fusion	Excellent
	P + C	Ortho or small esophoria

8. **Strabismus fixus**
    a. *Additional history:*
        Longstanding ET

    b. *Test:*   *Indicates:*

Forced ductions	Positive MR tightening
Measurements	Large ET, greater in R and L gaze
Versions/ductions	Decreased ABDuction, fixed ADDuction
Vision	Must cross-fixate and turn head to see

9. **Divergence paralysis**
    a. *Additional history:*
        General health: Normal intracranial pressure
        Infections, parasites, and travel abroad
        Possible trauma

    b. *Test:*   *Indicates:*

Divergence amplitudes	Nearly nonexistent
Versions/ductions	Full, ABDuction okay
Diplopia testing	Uncrossed, worse at distance
Measurements	Comitant esodeviation D>N
Fusion	May fuse at near
Vision	Equal

10. **Accommodative effort syndrome**
    a. *Additional history:*
        Near asthenopia, blurring, or diplopia

    b. *Test:*   *Indicates:*

Near point of accommodation (NPA)	Normal
P + C	E', possible E(T)'
Divergence amplitudes	Poor
Plus lenses for near	Helps relieve symptoms

(continued)

Table 7-1 (continued)

Esodeviations

11. Pseudo ET

   a. *Additional History:*

      Onset: usually since birth

      Appears incomitant

	Test:	*Indicates:*
b.	Hirschberg/cover-uncover/cross-cover	No deviation
	External	Frequently has epicanthal folds
	Angle kappa	Negative
	Fusion	Excellent, no suppression
	Versions/ductions	Appears to have increasing ET to right and left gaze because of epicanthal folds
	Divergence amplitudes	Intact

Table 7-2

Decreased ABDuction

1. Duane retraction syndrome type 1 (see Table 7-1.4)
2. CN VI palsy (see Table 7-1.3)
3. Infantile ET (see Table 7-1.1)
4. Nystagmus compensation syndrome (see Table 7-1.6)
5. Strabismus fixus (see Table 7-1.8)
6. Moebius syndrome (see Table 7-1.3)
7. Duane retraction syndrome type 3 (see Table 7-8)
8. Myasthenia gravis (see Table 7-1.3)

Table 7-3

Exodeviations

1. **Basic, divergence excess type, convergence insufficiency type**
   a. *Additional history:*
      Intermittency
      Worse at distance or near
      Worse with fatigue, illness

   b. *Test:*   *Indicates:*
      Fusion   Usually excellent
      Measurements   Exodeviation, usually comitant
      Vision   Equal
      Convergence amplitudes   Poor fusional convergence amps

2. **Infantile XT**
   a. *Additional history:*
      Present since birth
      Eye preference

   b. *Test:*   *Indicates:*
      Vision   Decreased in nonpreferred eye
      Health of eyes   No specific ocular disease
      Measurements   Usually large comitant XT

3. **MR palsy/CN III palsy**
   a. *Additional history:*
      Present since birth if congenital
      Severe trauma
      General health: possible headaches,
         myasthenia gravis
      Other signs: ipsilateral ptosis, mydriasis,
         cycloplegia, hypodeviation, contralateral
         body paralysis (Benedikt's syndrome)

   b. *Test:*   *Indicates:*
      Versions/ductions   Decreased ADDuction
      Measurements   Incomitant exodeviation, greater in
                                         ADDuction

      Measure with OD, OS fix   Primary and secondary deviation
      Vision   Possible amblyopia, cycloplegia
      Head position   Present if to attain fusion

4. **Duane retraction syndrome type 2**
   a. *Additional history:*
      No trauma
      Lid fissure changes with gaze
      Abnormal head position
      Present since birth

(continued)

Table 7-3 (continued)

Exodeviations

4. **Duane retraction syndrome type 2 (continued)**

b. *Test:*	*Indicates:*
Versions/ductions	Decreased ADDuction with lid narrowing, ABDuction okay
Head position	Needed to achieve fusion
Fusion with head position	Often present
Vision	Possible amblyopia

5. **Blind eye**

   a. *Additional history:*
   Age of blindness in one eye (if over 7, likely to drift exo)
   Constant nonalternating XT

b. *Test:*	*Indicates:*
Vision	Blind eye
Krimsky measurements	Fairly comitant XT

6. **Consecutive XT**

   a. *Additional history:*
   Previous surgery for ET

b. *Test:*	*Indicates:*
Measurements	XT
Fusion	Diplopia or suppression/ARC

7. **Cranial-facial anomalies**

   a. *Additional history:*
   Apert syndrome[2]
   Crouzon disease[2]

b. *Test:*	*Indicates:*
Measurements	Large VXT, RHT in left gaze, LHT in right gaze
Versions/ductions	IO overaction, SO underaction
External	Bilateral exophthalmos (Crouzon)
Refraction	Astigmatism (Apert)
	Progressive hyperopia (Crouzon)
Head scan	Globe rotated in orbit

8. **Convergence paralysis**

   a. *Additional history:*
   Trauma
   General health: Possible recent neurological condition

(continued)

Table 7-3 (continued)

Exodeviations

8.   Convergence paralysis (continued)

    b.   Test:

Convergence amplitudes	Nearly nonexistent
Measurements	Comitant exodeviation N>D
Versions/ductions	Full
Diplopia	Crossed, worse at near
Fusion	Distance only
Vision	Equal

Indicates:

9.   Internuclear ophthalmoplegia (INO)

    a.   Additional history:

        Bilateral: Systemic multiple sclerosis

        Unilateral: Vascular accident, inflammation, infection, tumor in brainstem, possible myasthenia gravis

    b.   Test: *Indicates:*

Versions/ductions	Decreased ADDuction with jerk nystagmus in ABDucted eye
Convergence amplitudes	Intact convergence

10.   Pseudo XT

    a.   Additional history:

        Constant

    b.   Test: *Indicates:*

Krimsky/cover-uncover	No eye deviation
Fusion	Excellent, no suppression
Angle kappa	Positive
Funduscopy	May have retinopathy of prematurity with temporally dragged fovea

Table 7-4

Decreased ADDuction

1.   Duane retraction syndrome type 2 (see Table 7-3.4)
2.   CN III palsy, MR palsy (see Tables 7-3.3, 7-7.5)
3.   Internuclear ophthalmoplegia (INO) (see Table 7-3.9)
4.   Myasthenia gravis (see Table 7-3.3, 7-3.9)

Table 7-5

Hyperdeviations

1. **Isolated cyclovertical muscle palsy (SO most common)**

   a. *Additional history:*

   Trauma, may be mild

   Head tilt, turn

   Combined horizontal and vertical diplopia

   Diplopia/asthenopia worse to right and left

   Myasthenia gravis   *Indicates:*

   Old photographs   Old head tilt if congenital/longstanding

   External inspection   Facial slant if congenital/longstanding
        (horizontal lines of brows and lips are
        not parallel)

   b. *Test:*   *Indicates:*

   Fusion with head position   Usually fuses

   P + C, nine positions   Incomitant HT

   3ST   Isolates EOM palsy

   Versions/ductions   SO—May show underactive SO,
        overactive IO, inhibitional palsy
        of contralateral (IPC) SR

                                              IO—May show underactive IO,
        overactive SO, IPC IR

         SR—May show underactive SR,
        overactive IR, IPC SO

         IR—May show underactive IR,
        overactive SR, IPC IO

   Vertical amplitudes   May exist if congenital/longstanding
        No vertical amps if recent onset

   Subjective torsion   May exist if recent onset
        SO, SR-extorsion
        IO, IR-intorsion

2. **DVD**

   a. *Additional history:*

   Associated with congenital/infantile ET

   One or both eyes go up, neither eye ever goes
      hypotropic

   Intermittent HT, either eye

   b. *Test:*   *Indicates:*

   Cover-uncover   Either eye elevates under cover without
        associated hypodeviation of the fellow
        eye

   P + C   Difficult to measure, variable

   Versions/ductions   Rule out IO overaction as "cause"

(continued)

Table 7-5 (continued)
Hyperdeviations

3. Brown syndrome

  a. Additional history:

Trauma to trochlear region of globe

Sinus, orbital surgery

Juvenile rheumatoid arthritis

Present since birth if congenital

b. Test:	*Indicates:*
Version/ductions	No elevation of globe in ADDuction
	Eye elevates easily in ABDuction
Forced ductions	Restriction of globe up and in
Fusion	Often fuses in downgaze
Vision	Possible amblyopia
Krimsky	Hypotropia of affected eye when up and in

4. Blowout fracture

  a. Additional history:

Blunt trauma-orbital fracture

Diplopia/discomfort often worse in upgaze

b. Test:	*Indicates:*
Ductions/versions	Hypotropia worsens toward upgaze
	Restrictions of ductions: upgaze
	may be down, right, or left gaze
Forced ductions	Restriction of globe, usually upgaze
X-ray/CT scan	Orbital fracture, frequently floor or nasal
	wall
Diplopia field	Often has region of single binocular
	vision
Exophthalmometry	Affected eye often enophthalmic

5. Double elevator palsy (DEP)

  a. Additional history:

Present since birth

Ptosis on affected side

Chin up head position

No trauma

b. Test:	*Indicates:*
Fusion with chin up	Possible fusion
Versions/ductions	Constant hypotropia of affected eye
Forced ductions	No restrictions of elevation unless very
	longstanding
External	Pseudo ptosis on affected side

(continued)

Table 7-5 (continued)

Hyperdeviations

6. Graves' ophthalmopathy

   a. Additional history:
   Thyroid dysfunction in past or present

   b. Test: *Indicates:*
   Ductions/versions   Restriction of upgaze (IR), lateral gaze
                                               (MR), or any EOM
   Forced ductions   Positive for restriction
   Fusion with head position   May have fusion
   Diplopia   Variable vertical > horizontal and torsional

7. Pseudo HT

   a. Additional history:
   Previous EOM or lid surgery

   b. Test: *Indicates:*
   Cover-uncover   No deviation
   Lift lid   Appearance of HT disappears
   Assess pupils   Possible asymmetry
   External photography   No deviation by light reflex

Table 7-6

True Hypodeviations

1. Brown syndrome (see Table 7-5.3)
2. Double elevator palsy (see Table 7-5.5)
3. Blowout fracture (see Table 7-5.4)
4. Restrictive thyroid eye disease (Graves') (see Table 7-5.6)

Table 7-7

Decreased Elevation

1. **Thyroid ophthalmopathy (see Table 7-5.6)**
2. **Brown syndrome (see Table 7-5.3)**
3. **Blowout fracture (see Table 7-5.4)**
4. **Double elevator palsy (see Table 7-5.5)**
5. **Myasthenia gravis (see Table 7-5.1)**
6. **CN III palsy**
   a. *Additional history:*
      Ptosis, mydriasis, decreased elevation, and
         ADDuction
      Trauma possible
      Present since birth if congenital
      Diabetes in adult

b. *Test:*	*Indicates:*
Versions/ductions	Absent elevation and ADDuction
Forced ductions	No restrictions unless very longstanding
Lid assessment	Ptosis, may be complete
Pupil assessment	No reaction to light or accommodation, unless diabetic
Vision/refraction	Cyclopleged, unless diabetic
Krimsky	Incomitance, often never ortho
ABDuction (LR)	Intact
Depression, intorsion (SO)	Intact

Table 7-8

Decreased Ductions

1. **Duane retraction syndrome type 1 (see Table 7-1.4)**
2. **Duane retraction syndrome type 2 (see Table 7-3.4)**
3. **Duane retraction syndrome type 3**
   a. *Additional history:*
      No trauma
      Lid fissure changes with gaze
      Present since birth

b. *Test:*	*Indicates:*
Versions/ductions	Absent ABDuction and ADDuction
	Enophthalmos during attempted ADDuction with narrowing of lid fissure

4. **Cyclovertical muscle palsy (see Table 7-5.1)**
5. **Brown syndrome (see Table 7-5.3)**
6. **Blowout fracture (see Table 7-5.4)**
7. **Thyroid ophthalmopathy (see Table 7-5.6)**
8. **Strabismus fixus (see Table 7-1.8)**

Table 7-9

Abnormal Head Position

1. **Congenital torticollis**
   a. *Additional history:*
      Present since able to hold head up unassisted
         (approximately 6 months of age)
      No eye turn or nystagmus ever seen
   b. *Test:*   *Indicates:*
      Prolonged occlusion   Head position persists
      EOM exam   No motility disturbance
      Force head tilt to opposite side   No hyperdeviation seen (no SO palsy)

2. **Congenital nystagmus**
   a. *Additional history:*
      Horizontal jerk nystagmus seen without head
         position
      Nystagmus damps during near fixation
      Present since birth
   b. *Test:*   *Indicates:*
      Binocular, monocular vision   Usually better binocularly
      Versions/ductions   Nystagmus worse away from null point
      Assess nystagmus, D + N   Usually less at near

3. **CN IV palsy (see Table 7-5.1)**

4. **Duane retraction syndrome types 1, 2, 3 (see Tables 7-1.4, 7-3.4, 7-8.3)**

5. **Nystagmus compensation syndrome (see Table 7-1.6)**

6. **Strabismus fixus (see Table 7-1.8)**

7. **Graves' ophthalmopathy (see Table 7-5.6)**

8. **Uncorrected refractive error**
   a. *Additional history:*
      Child observed squinting
      Child observed with chin down head position
   b. *Test:*   *Indicates:*
      Vision   Squints in order to see better
                                                 Chin down persists monocularly
      Refractive error   Reduces squinting on head position

Table 7-10

Diplopia

1. **Uncorrected refractive error causing blur**
    a. *Additional history:*
        Images very close together
        Possibly more than two images per eye
    b. *Test:*   *Indicates:*
        Refraction   Frequent astigmatism, blur disappears
                                                     with proper refractive correction

        Pinhole   Second image disappears

2. **Monocular diplopia**
    a. *Additional history:*
        Diplopia persists in one or both eyes with
            occlusion
        Extra image(s) may be blurred or smeared
        Injury to cornea/lens causing scarring
        Retinal injury, laser
        Bifocal line obstructing visual axis
    b. *Test:*   *Indicates:*
        Monocular occlusion   Diplopia persists
        Health of eye   Organic cause of diplopia
                                                     Rule out cataract or corneal opacity
        Refraction   Frequent astigmatism

True Binocular Diplopias

3. **Decompensated phoria now tropic**
    a. *Additional history:*
        Previous intermittent tropia with diplopia
    b. *Test:*   *Indicates:*
        Fusion with deviation corrected   Usually fuses
        P + C   Often comitant, usually XT or HT
        Fusion potential   Usually excellent

4. **EOM palsy (see Tables 7-1.3, 7-3.3, 7-5.1)**

5. **Newly noticed diplopia from longstanding condition**
    a. *Additional history:*
        Brown syndrome (see Table 7-5)
        Duane retraction syndrome types 1, 2, 3
            (see Tables 7-1.4, 7-3.4, 7-8.3)
        Thyroid ophthalmopathy (see Table 7-5.6)
        Blowout fracture (see Table 7-5.4)
        Has the patient ever looked into that field
            of gaze before? (Probably not)

(continued)

Table 7-10 (continued)

Diplopia

6. Secondary to restrictive strabismus

    a.   *Additional history:*

        Thyroid ophthalmopathy (see Table 7-5.6)

        Brown syndrome (see Table 7-5.3)

        Duane retraction syndrome types 1, 2, 3

            (see Tables 7-1.4, 7-3.4, 7-8.3)

        If the strabismus had been present since

            childhood, has the patient ever looked into

            that field of gaze before? (Probably not)

7.   **Divergence paralysis (see Table 7-1.9)**

8.   **Convergence paralysis (see Table 7-3.8)**

9.   **Intractable diplopia**

    a.   *Additional history:*

        Previous antisuppression exercises

        Trauma

        Previous strabismus surgery

b. *Test:*	*Indicates:*
Fusion potential	None
Occlusion	No diplopia
Retinal correspondence	Often abnormal, paradoxical

10. **Paradoxical diplopia**

    a.   *Additional history:*

        Previous strabismus surgery

        Consecutive tropia

b. *Test:*	*Indicates:*
Retinal correspondence	ARC

11. **Glasses-induced**

    a.   *Additional history:*

        New glasses

        New bifocal

        Aphakic correction

        Glasses recently adjusted

        Diplopia disappears with glasses removed

        Diplopia is typically vertical but may be uncrossed

b. *Test:*	*Indicates:*
Check for prism in glasses	Optical center misalignment creating prism, typically vertical or base-in
Check height of bifocal	May be asymmetric

Table 7-11

Near Vision Problems

1. **Convergence insufficiency**
    a. *Additional history:*
        Blurring while reading/near work or prolonged
            distance fixation
        Occasional horizontal diplopia
        Difficulty changing from N to D or D to N fixation
        Headaches after using eyes; never upon awakening

    b. *Test:*   *Indicates:*
        Fusion   Normal stereopsis
        P + C   May have small to large exo, eso, or may
                                                 be ortho
                                             Often has congenital SO palsy
        Fusional amplitudes   Poor fusional amplitudes for visual
                                                 demands, uses accommodative
                                                 convergence, poor recovery/jump point
        Prolonged occlusion   Symptoms completely disappear

2. **Presbyopia**
    a. *Additional history:*
        40+ years old
        Previous hyperopic correction
        Older myope who was recently fit with
            contact lenses for the first time
        Older hyperope who was recently switched
            from contact lenses to full-time glasses

    b. *Test:*   *Indicates:*
        Cycloplegic refraction   Possibly overminused or has latent
                                                 hyperopia
        NPA, cc   Should be normal for age

3. **Systemic convergence insufficiency**
    a. *Additional history:*
        Trauma
        Illness: Encephalitis, drug intoxication,
            mononucleosis[1]
        Increasing diplopia and blurring with near vision

    b. *Test:*   *Indicates:*
        Convergence   Convergence insufficiency
        NPA   Severely decreased and often fixed
        Plus lenses   Improves near vision
        Near P + C   Constant XT at N requiring BI prism for
                                                 fusion

(continued)

Table 7-11 (continued)

Near Vision Problems

4.   Convergence paralysis (see Table 7-3.8)

5.   Divergence paralysis (see Table 7-1.9)

6.   Accommodative spasm

    a.   Additional history:
        Possible psychogenesis
        Severe distance blurring after near fixation

    b.   Test: *Indicates:*

Test:	Indicates:
Distance VA	Usually worse than 20/200
Manifest refraction	Up to 8 to 10 D myopia
Cycloplegic refraction	High myopia disappears

7.   Accommodative effort syndrome (see Table 7-1.10)

8.   Juvenile presbyopia

    a.   Additional history:
        Drug use
        History of hysteria
        Symptoms of presbyopia, except age is
            much younger

    b.   Test: *Indicates:*

Test:	Indicates:
Near vision	Decreased
P + C	Insignificant eye turn
NPA	Decreased for age
Plus lenses for near	Relieves symptoms
Cycloplegic refraction	Minimal refractive error

9.   CN IV palsy (SO palsy) (see Table 7-5.1)

    a.   Additional history:
        Asthenopia, diplopia increases in reading position

Table 7-12

Pseudostrabismus

1. **Prominent epicanthal folds appear (ET) (see Table 7-1.11)**

2. **Narrow lateral canthi appears (XT)**

3. **Angle kappa**
   Positive appears (XT) (see Table 7-3.9)
   Negative (ET) (see Table 7-1.11)

4. **Ectopic macula**
   a. *Additional history:*
       Previous retinal problems or surgery
   b. *Test:*   *Indicates:*
       Funduscopy   Displaced macula

5. **Anisocoria**
   a. *Additional history:*
       May be associated with mild ptosis with miotic
           pupil (Horner syndrome)
       May or may not have heterochromia (congenital
           Horner syndrome has heterochromia)
       May or may not have facial anhydrosis (absence
           of perspiration)
       Trauma
       CN III palsy
   b. *Test:*   *Indicates:*
       Pupil evaluation   Anisocoria
       Cover-uncover   No eye deviation
       Fusion   Normal

6. **Exophthalmos (see Table 7-13)**

Table 7-13

Exophthalmos

1. **Graves' ophthalmopathy**
   a. *Additional history:*
      Proptosis not present years ago
      Thyroid disease
      Diplopia, particularly in upgaze
      May be both eyes, but asymmetrical
   b. *Test:*   *Indicates:*
      Exophthalmometry   Either greater than 22 mm or difference
                                         between eyes >2 mm
      Lid fissure height   May be greater on side of proptosis

2. **Orbital tumors: Lymphoma, malignant melanoma, rhabdomyosarcoma, retinoblastoma, neurofibroma, glioma, dermoid, lacrimal gland tumor, carcinoma, mucocele**
   a. *Additional history:*
      May be sudden onset
      May be any age, frequently children
      Associated with other illness
   b. *Test:*   *Indicates:*
      Exophthalmometry   Exophthalmos
      CT scan, B scan   Orbital mass

3. **Inflammations: Pseudotumor, myositis**
   a. *Additional history:*
      Pain
      Ophthalmoplegia

4. **Infections: Orbital cellulitis**
   a. *Additional history:*
      Sudden onset, worsens quickly
      Hot eye
      Monocular
      Usually young child
   b. *Test:*   *Indicates:*
      CT scan   Orbital involvement
      General health   Sick child/fever/malaise

(continued)

Table 7-13 (continued)
Exophthalmos

5. **Vascular disorders: Orbital varix, cavernous sinus thrombosis, pulsating exophthalmos**

   a. *Additional history:*

     Eye bulges when baby cries (varix)

     Previous orbital infection (thrombosis)

     Neurofibromatosis

   b. *Test:*   *Indicates:*

     Orbital venography   A-V malformation

     View patient from side   Pulsating exophthalmos visible

6. **Orbital anomalies: Crouzon syndrome, Apert syndrome[2]**

7. **Enophthalmos of contralateral eye**

   a. *Additional history:*

     Blowout fracture

     Blind, phthisical eye

   b. *Test:*   *Indicates:*

     Exophthalmometry   Enophthalmos of contralateral eye

8. **Pseudoexophthalmos**

   a. *Additional history:*

     Old photographs

     Unilateral lid retraction or ptosis

     Large eye due to buphthalmos (juvenile glaucoma), axial myopia, or staphyloma

     True enophthalmos of contralateral eye

   b. *Test:*   *Indicates:*

     Exophthalmometry   Normal

Table 7-14
Enophthalmos

1. Blowout fracture (see Table 7-5.4)
2. Phthisis bulbi (see Table 7-13.7)
3. Pseudo-real exophthalmos of contralateral eye (see Table 7-13)

References

1. Raskind RH. Problems at the reading distance. *Am Orthopt J.* 1976;26:53-59.
2. Harley RD. *Pediatric Ophthalmology.* Philadelphia, PA: WB Saunders; 1975.

Chapter 8

Syndromes With Ocular Manifestations

KEY POINTS

- Syndromes may be congenital (present at birth) yet not be apparent until later in life.

- Some syndromes develop over time and, therefore, are not considered congenital.

- Early diagnosis of a syndrome is essential so that proper treatment can be initiated.

A syndrome is a constellation of characteristic findings. Once the syndrome is identified, the characteristics of it can be found in the patient. Early diagnosis of a syndrome helps initiate proper treatment and, in some cases, can help other clinicians identify additional problems in the patient's health. Some typical syndromes are often found when examining children and adults with strabismus.

Duane Retraction Syndrome—Co-Contraction Syndrome

Duane retraction syndrome is a horizontal deviation that is present at birth and varies in primary, right, and left gazes. It is thought to be caused by a misfiring, or true cofiring, of the medial rectus (MR) and lateral rectus (LR). The patient is often ortho near or in the primary position may fuse and may have equal vision in each eye. Duane syndrome type 1 causes an increasingly larger esotropia (ET) to the ABDucting side. In primary position, a small ET is often present, but the patient may be ortho. Type 2 causes an increasingly larger exotropia (XT) to the ADDucting side. Type 3 is decreased ABDuction and ADDuction of the eye so that the ET increases to the ABDucting side and the XT increases to the ADDucting side. All three types result in both narrowing of the lid fissure and globe retraction when ADDuction is attempted. Duane syndrome may be bilateral. For unknown reasons, Duane syndrome is predominantly found in females and most commonly affects the left eye (Table 8-1).

The physiology of Duane syndrome is as follows: when ABDuction of the affected eye is attempted, no innervation goes to the LR, so the eye does not go fully into ABDuction. The eyelid fissure often widens. When ADDuction is attempted, both the MR and LR are innervated simultaneously (not in accordance with Sherrington's law of reciprocal innervation), and the eye is pulled back into the orbit, causing narrowing of the palpebral fissure. The globe retraction is best viewed from the side as the eye is directed to go from ABDuction into ADDuction. ADDuction itself may be slightly deficient. Excessive upshooting or downshooting of the affected eye may occur during attempted ADDuction. This mimics an overactive inferior oblique or superior oblique but is actually due to the extremely tight lateral rectus as it inappropriately contracts during attempted ADDuction. The eyeball itself slips up or down against the lateral rectus.

When fusion can often be attained without significant head positioning, surgery is usually not necessary. If there is a cumbersome head position, surgery becomes necessary to reduce it. There is the risk of developing amblyopia, and this should be evaluated and treated appropriately in the young child. To establish strong fusion, patients with Duane syndrome should be encouraged to use their head position. Table 8-2 lists the tests that should be done on a patient with Duane syndrome.

Goldenhar Syndrome

Children with Goldenhar syndrome have both an ocular dermoid (frequently limbal epibulbar) and external ear deformities ranging from preauricular skin tags (extra pieces of skin on their face just in front of their ear) to no external ear at all. Other ocular findings include Duane syndrome and lid, iris, or choroidal colobomas. Children with Goldenhar syndrome may be deaf, or they may have vertebral anomalies. Because the dermoid may cause corneal astigmatism, the patient must be refracted at every visit. The patient should be watched for the development of ambloypia.[1]

Table 8-1

Duane Syndrome: All three types have narrowing of lid fissure with globe retraction during attempted ADDuction

Type 1: Decreased ABDuction
Type 2: Decreased ADDuction
Type 3: Decreased ABDuction and ADDuction

Table 8-2

Tests for Duane Syndrome	Results
Stereopsis/fusion	Usually intact with head position
P + C: In primary position	Small tropia, often ET
and secondary positions	Incomitance
Versions	Decreased ABDuction (type 1), ADDuction (type 2), or both (type 3)
	Lid fissure narrowing in ADDuction
Vision	Rule out amblyopia
Other	Note any head position; look at old pictures

Brown Syndrome—Superior Oblique Tendon Sheath Syndrome

Brown syndrome is a mechanical restriction preventing free passage of the superior oblique (SO) through its trochlea when the eye looks up and in. There appears to be decreased elevation in ADDuction by duction testing (the inferior oblique [IO] appears weak). The patient may have a chin-up head position to put the eyes into fusional range in downgaze. Although Brown syndrome is often congenital (and monocular), it may be acquired through damage—either traumatic or iatrogenic—to the trochlea itself or to the portion of the SO that glides through the trochlea. Although it usually presents as a clear clinical picture, positive forced duction testing definitely confirms the diagnosis.

In Brown syndrome, the eyes are often straight in the primary position, so fusion is often present and amblyopia uncommon. A child who frequently looks up in the IO's field on the affected side will suppress the extra image. The child who does not often look into that field will not develop suppression and will be diplopic in that field of gaze as an adult. Table 8-3 lists the tests that should be performed on a patient with Brown syndrome.

Some children with juvenile rheumatoid arthritis (JRA) have a SO "click" syndrome. When ductions or forced ductions are performed, the eye will not elevate in ADDuction at first. But with continued attempts, the SO literally clicks through the obstruction and the eye pops up into position. For this reason, any child with new onset of Brown syndrome should be evaluated for JRA.[2]

Superior Oblique Myokymia

SO myokymia is an intermittent twitching of the SO muscle. This results in an annoying quivering of the world as seen by that eye. The patient describes fine movement of the object of

Table 8-3	
Tests for Brown Syndrome	**Results**
P + C: Primary position	May be ortho
Secondary positions	Hypodeviation in upgaze
Tertiary positions	Hypotropia in ADDuction only
Head tilts	No EOM palsy
Versions	Limited elevation in ADDuction
Ductions	Limited elevation in ADDuction
Vision	Rule out amblyopia
Stereopsis/fusion	Often intact

Table 8-4	
Tests for Monofixation Syndrome	**Results**
Stereopsis	Less than 67 seconds of arc
Simultaneous P + C	Small constant esotropia (may be XT or vertical)
P + C	Larger phoria
Vision	Mild amblyopia
Refraction	Often anisometropic
4-diopter base-out test	Monocular suppression
Worth four-dot	Fusion at near
	Monocular suppression at distance
Bagolini lenses	Cross (fusion) with central scotoma

regard and can sometimes describe the vertical/torsional component of the deviation. Typically, the movement is caused by one eye, so closing that eye eliminates it. When the unaffected eye is closed, the motion is apparent. Like a lid twitch, SO myokymia usually goes away by itself but may require neurological medical intervention. The diagnosis is usually made through history, but an episode is best viewed at the slit lamp. Watch the iris crypts or conjunctival blood vessels, looking for quick intorsional movements of the globe.

Monofixation Syndrome

Monofixation syndrome has been called many different things but is most commonly described by saying that the patient is a monofixator. It is usually an esodeviation but also can be manifest as an exo-, hyper-, or hypodeviation. Monofixation may even be manifest in an ortho patient. The manifest deviation never exceeds 8 prism diopters (PD) of either ET or XT or more than 3 PD of hyper- or hypotropia.

This syndrome is characterized by mild amblyopia—as little as a half line difference—and by fovea/central suppression of the affected eye on fusion tests such as the stereo test, Worth four-dot, or the 4-diopter base-out test. Table 8-4 lists tests and typical findings in a patient with monofixational syndrome. The eye turn in monofixation syndrome is not noticed by casual observation and goes undetected by patients, parents, and careless examiners. Ordinarily, there is a larger deviation that can be measured by alternate prism and cross (P + C) cover, and this is often the tip-off to the diagnosis. For example, during a cover–uncover test, a very small tropia (<8 PD) is noted. While measuring this tropia, the deviation builds larger and larger (up to 30 PD). When this happens, go back and look more carefully for a small constant tropia and for amblyopia and suppression of the tropic eye to make the diagnosis.

The 4-diopter base-out test for suppression/fusion is an objective test that helps determine eye preference by identifying central suppression. It also suggests the presence of sensory fusion because of the existence of fine motor fusion. In a normal patient who is straight and fusing, a small base-out prism introduced to either eye will ultimately cause a vergence movement. This is because the base-out prism induces a small exodeviation (with crossed diplopia), so a small convergence movement will be necessary to fixate bifoveally again. A small (4 PD) prism is used because almost all fusing patients are able to converge 4 PD, yet it provides enough movement of the eye for the examiner to observe.

A patient who suppresses foveally will not be able to tell when the 4 PD base-out prism is introduced. This is because the prism will cause the image on the retina to move only a small amount (only 4 D worth). The image will still fall within the eye's small suppression scotoma. The image over the suppressing eye can be caused to move in one of two ways. First, placing the prism directly over the suppressing eye will cause the image to move, but since the movement of the image is not perceived, the eye will make no attempt to refixate. Neither eye will move when the prism is placed over the suppressing eye. The second way to move the image is by placing the prism over the habitually fixing eye, which causes the retinal image to move off of the fovea. The fixing eye will ordinarily move inward (in the direction of the prism's apex) so as to pick up fixation. The other suppressing eye will move (in a version) with the fixing eye, but the retinal image continues to move within its suppression region, so no convergence movement is made. This would indicate suppression in the eye that did not converge.

The 4-diopter base-out prism test is extremely useful, as it is one of the few fusion tests that is purely objective. Patients cannot feign suppression when they do not have it or elicit a fusion response if one eye is suppressing. Practice this test and imagine how the eyes would respond if one eye was completely blind. The response to the introduction of the prism is the same whether the eye is blind or has a small suppression scotoma and 20/20 -3 vision. Also, you might practice this test using a 6-diopter prism so that the response is easier to see. Of course, to gain experience, practice this test on cooperative adults with and without equal vision.

While a patient with monofixation syndrome does not have bifoveal fusion, some gross peripheral fusion is present with a cosmetically acceptable eye turn. This fusion is demonstrated with the Bagolini lenses, which are two plano lenses with fine striations that cause a light fixation to appear as a line. When the patient with monofixation syndrome is presented with the Bagolini lenses, he or she will report seeing a cross, which indicates fusion in conjunction with the small tropia, but with a small gap in the center of one line that corresponds to the small suppression scotoma. Most monofixators require no treatment except if significant amblyopia is found in a child of treatable age. Many monofixators are anisometropic amblyopes and benefit from a balanced prescription. Some older patients may decompensate from their small monofixational state into their larger deviation. The patient may develop diplopia once his or her deviation is larger since the image now falls outside of the small suppression scotoma, causing him or her to become suddenly symptomatic. Establishing that the patient is actually a longstanding monofixator who has just decompensated can save everyone the cost and worry of a neurological examination to find other causes in an adult with a sudden ET.

Moebius Syndrome

Moebius syndrome is a unilateral or bilateral congenital syndrome in which a CN VI (abducens nerve) and CN VII (facial nerve) palsy combine, causing and ET with limited ABDuction and an inability to form facial expressions (or suck or chew well). An inability to completely close the eyelids may also result. Vertical movement of the eyes is unaffected. The extreme ET requires surgical treatment aimed at moving at least one eye to the primary position, thus enabling the patient to fixate without a large face turn. Young patients must be monitored for amblyopia.[3]

Gradenigo Syndrome

Gradenigo syndrome is a unilateral CN VI palsy caused by a middle ear infection. There is pain on the affected side of the face, possibly accompanied by partial or total hearing loss. Usually the CN VI and ET are spontaneously resolved with treatment of the ear infection. During the ET, amblyopia and tightening of the MR muscles may be prevented with occlusion.[4]

Accommodative Effort Syndrome

This is a rare phenomenon resulting in a small esophoria at near and asthenopic symptoms while reading. The monocular near point of accommodation (NPA) is normal, but accommodation is reduced when measured binocularly. There are poor amplitudes of relative fusion divergence but, as would be expected, increased amplitudes of accommodative convergence. Blurred vision during near fixation is caused by the patient's effort to have comfortable single binocular vision. The blurring is caused by relaxed accommodation, which decreases the accompanying accommodative convergence.[5]

Horner Syndrome

The combination of ptosis, miosis, and anhydrosis indicates Horner syndrome. There is an interruption of the sympathetic fibers that ordinarily dilate the pupil (so it is slightly miotic), raise the Mueller's lid muscle (so the lid is slightly lower), and may or may not affect perspiration of the face on that side (so that side of the face may be appreciably drier). New onset of Horner syndrome may be caused by trauma or lung lesions. Congenital Horner syndrome interrupts the progressive color changes that occur in the iris during infancy. The affected iris is lighter in color, producing heterochromia. Heterochromia in a patient with Horner syndrome indicates that the condition is congenital and not a new onset, which would require further systemic work-up.

Nystagmus Compensation Syndrome

Nystagmus compensation syndrome (NCS) causes a large ET that becomes apparent shortly after birth, so it is often mistaken for infantile ET. It is thought to be caused by jerk nystagmus, present only with the eye in ABDuction. As a compensation to improve vision, both eyes are kept in ADDuction. Since neither eye can be out of ADDuction without nystagmus, cross-fixation with a head turn results. NCS does look similar to infantile ET, except that jerk nystagmus is present when either eye moves past the midline into ABDuction. Parents frequently never see the nystagmus.

The tip-off leading to a diagnosis of NCS occurs when quantifying the child's eye turn by Krimsky measurements. The correcting base-out prism neutralizes the manifest deviation and forces one eye to the midline. Immediately, either nystagmus is evident or the child overconverges again, and large ET still exists despite the correcting base-out prism. Treatment is surgical.[6]

Marcus Gunn Jaw Winking Syndrome

Generally, this is a diagnosis that parents make for you; they can describe it so well that you could suspect it over the phone without ever seeing the child. The baby may or may not have ptosis, but the lid position varies (or winks) when the baby sucks or moves his or her jaw. Chewing, yawning, or smiling may also cause the lid to move. This syndrome is caused by a congenital miswiring of the nerves to the lid and maxilla, causing the levator muscle to work when the jaw is moving. Like any young ptosis patient, amblyopia is a concern. Cosmesis becomes more of a problem when the child gets older. Lid surgery is necessary if the lid is covering the visual axis. The response to typical lid surgery is variable since the nerve to the lid is still faulty regardless of what has surgically been done. Patients, however, usually learn to hold their jaw just so as to make the one lid match the other.

Marfan Syndrome

Marfan syndrome is characterized by four findings—dislocation of the crystalline lens, heart problems (which can be life threatening), musculoskeletal abnormalities (exhibited by unusually tall individuals with long limbs and long, double-jointed fingers), and a family history of Marfan syndrome. The absence of zonules results in the dislocation of the lenses. Initially, this causes extremely distorted and varying refractive errors and, later, aphakic refractive errors once the lens is completely out of the visual axis. Older patients may benefit from lens extraction and intraocular lens placement, but subsequent problems with raised intraocular pressure may result.[7]

Apert and Crouzon Syndromes

These two craniofacial syndromes are congenital syndromes that result in abnormal closure of the infant's cranial sutures.[8] Abnormally shaped skulls result. Patients with Crouzon syndrome have unusually shallow orbits, resulting in progressively shorter eyes and hyperopia. Patients with Apert syndrome have webbed fingers and toes, which requires surgery to correct. Both types of patients have hypertelorism and have been found to have large exodeviations. They may have very large V pattern exodeviations that mimic bilateral SO palsies. In fact, the globes and, therefore, muscle insertions are rotated within the abnormal orbits. Because of the cranial abnormalities, fitting glasses properly is difficult and may require modifying an adult frame for a child.

Down Syndrome—Trisomy 21

Children with Down syndrome frequently have ocular abnormalities. A significant number of these children will have strabismus, most frequently ET. A and V patterns with head positioning are also common, so measurements in up- and downgaze are imperative in their pediatric ophthalmology work-up. Brushfield's spots in the iris, blepharitis, latent nystagmus, cataracts, keratoconus, and significant refractive errors are all reported in Down syndrome.[9] Optical correction may be challenging and requires knowledgeable ophthalmic dispensers.

References

1. Harley RD. *Pediatric Ophthalmology*. Philadelphia, PA: WB Saunders; 1975;17:211-212.

2. Killiam P, McClain B, Lawless O. Brown's syndrome—an unusual manifestation of rheumatoid arthritis. *Arthritis Rheum*. 1977;20:5.

3. Harley RD. *Pediatric Ophthalmology*. Philadelphia, PA: WB Saunders; 1975;162-163.

4. Harley RD. *Pediatric Ophthalmology*. Philadelphia, PA: WB Saunders; 1975;458.

5. Hurtt J, Rasicovici A, Windsor CE. *Comprehensive Review of Orthoptics and Ocular Motility*. 2nd ed. St. Louis, MO: CV Mosby; 1977:145.

6. Frank JW. Diagnostic signs in the nystagmus compensation syndrome. *J Pediatr Ophthalmol Strabismus*. 1979;16(5):317-320.

7. Harley RD. *Pediatric Ophthalmology*. Philadelphia, PA: WB Saunders; 1975:46,387.

8. Harley RD. *Pediatric Ophthalmology*. Philadelphia, PA: WB Saunders; 1975:360.

9. Harley RD. *Pediatric Ophthalmology*. Philadelphia, PA; WB Saunders; 1975:33.

Chapter 9

Nonsurgical Treatment of Strabismus

KEY POINTS

- Compliance for all treatment plans starts with patient education.

- Know your local optical shops and opticians.

- Amblyopia requires aggressive treatment.

- Fusing patients may benefit from exercises aimed at strengthening their amplitudes.

- Prisms should be used only to restore fusion.

Treatment of pediatric eye problems and adult strabismus really falls into two categories: what absolutely needs to be done and what is actually feasible. When deciding if the treatment is practical, one must take into consideration whether the patient is a wild 2 year old with parents/ guardians willing to take on the challenge or an adult who requires that our intervention results in a better outcome than what he or she started with!

Treatment of strabismic patients often involves three groups: the patient (who may be a child), the parent (who carries the guilt, the ability to do what is right, and the legal responsibility to make that decision), and the referring doctor (who sent the patient in the first place). Referring doctors, whether they are pediatricians or neurosurgeons, need to be educated about what is available for their patients. They will not send the patient unless they realize that there is a specialist who can do what would have been impossible in previous years. As always, education is the key.

Refractive Errors

Once a refractive error is discovered, it becomes necessary to determine if treating it is actu- ally needed. Not all −0.50 spherical myopes need to be corrected. The 3 year old probably does not need correction; the 20-year-old college student in a big auditorium copying information from a small monitor located a football field away certainly does. Mild anisometropia in a young child really does not need to be corrected if there is no amblyopia. A child with any anisometro- pia should have his or her vision watched carefully to detect amblyopia before it is irreversible, but glasses are not necessarily prescribed simply to avoid it. When the anisometropia is more extreme, there are new benefits to prescribing the correction that go beyond prophylactically treating amblyopia with glasses. The benefits include increased binocularity, which may not develop if the anisometropia is not balanced at a young age.

When glasses are prescribed for children, it is imperative to balance the two eyes. This means the correction must compensate for any anisometropia so that even if the full plus prescription is not given, the correction still allows each eye to receive a clear image at the same time. The full amount of astigmatism is corrected. Examples of balance prescriptions are shown in Table 9-1.

An adult with longstanding amblyopia, loss of binocularity, and anisometropia may suddenly become symptomatic if the full balanced prescription is given. Radical changes in adult prescrip- tions should be tried out first, either with loose lenses in the trial frame or by placing temporary Fresnel press-on lenses over the glasses. The "balance lens" that many anisometropic amblyopic adults have is rarely a lens that balances their true prescription. The balance lens is merely a lens that is similar to the other eye's prescription so that it does not cosmetically magnify or minify the eye. Giving an adult a true balanced prescription may not work if the patient is used to such a balance lens over the amblyopic eye.

Bifocal Adds

Bifocals are given to children for two main reasons: aphakia and high accommodative con- vergence/accommodation (AC/A) ratios.

Infants who have had a monocular congenital cataract removed are usually placed in con- tact lenses that correct them for near fixation (ie, they are overplussed by 2 to 3 diopters [D]). Because their world is close up within reach, this overcorrection that blurs them for distance and clears them for near works well. As they reach preschool age at 3 to 3.5 years, their visual

	Table 9-1		
	Examples of Balanced Prescriptions		
Cycloplegic		**Balanced RX**	
OD	+3.50 sph	OD	Plano sph
OS	+5.75 sph	OS	+2.25 sph
OD	+2.75 + 1.00 x 090	OD	+2.50 + 1.00 x 090
OS	+0.25 + 1.50 x 085	OS	PL + 1.50 x 085
OD	+0.50 + 3.50 x 050	OD	-0.25 + 3.50 x 050
OS	-1.00 + 4.25 x 160	OS	-1.75 + 4.25 x 160

needs require correction for both distance and near. At this point, the contact lens is prescribed for distance correction, and glasses are prescribed to give the child a bifocal segment add. The glasses may be plano for distance or could correct for any residual astigmatism not corrected by the contacts. Since aniseikonia is rarely a symptomatic issue in childhood aphakia, overplussing the contact lens and then compensating with excess minus in the distance spectacle correction is not necessary. In cases of microphthalmos, the contact lens can be adjusted so that a magnifying overcorrection improves the child's cosmesis. Also, wearing glasses may protect the lens from the increasingly active and interactive life of the preschooler.

The segment add used for an aphakic child is typically a traditional flat top initially, but may be a progressive style later. The segment height is placed uncharacteristically high (splitting the pupil) so that it will encourage the child to use the bifocal. Later, bifocals can be placed at a less distracting height, particularly once the child is doing board work.

High AC/A ratios also require a bifocal add, but for both eyes, in order to straighten the child's eyes at near fixation and permit fusion. Bifocals given to children with high AC/A ratios should be flat tops. A D-35 style is appropriate, as it is wide enough to encompass most of a young child's frame width (Figure 9-1).

Accommodative esotropia (ET) is corrected by wearing the full cycloplegic correction for distance; this may (in a normal AC/A ratio) or may not (as in a high AC/A ratio) fully correct the tendency to cross at near when the child accommodates 3 additional diopters in order to see clearly. When an ET at near persists despite wearing the full cycloplegic refraction, a near add is then prescribed, generally starting with +3.00. For practical purposes, both economic and treatment-wise, the bifocal add should be given at the time the first glasses are given.

So how could the clinician know if the child will need an add at the first visit? The measurements taken on any child who might have accommodative ET (which is any child with ET) must include the near measurements taken also with additional plus lenses. Dry retinoscopy provides a good estimate of the measurement of hyperopia, so the near measurement should be taken with the dry retinoscopy in place. If an ET still persists at near, then additional +1.00, +2.00, and ultimately +3.00 lenses should be tried while recording not just the size of the esodeviation but the fusional state (phoria versus tropia versus intermittency). While wearing those plus lenses in the office for a few moments really is not a fair judge of whether or not the glasses will ultimately work if the child is still esotropic, it does give the clinician valuable information when the plus lenses do straighten out the eyes. The lenses that decrease the near deviation into fusional range (converts an ET to an esophoria or orthophoria) are prescribed.

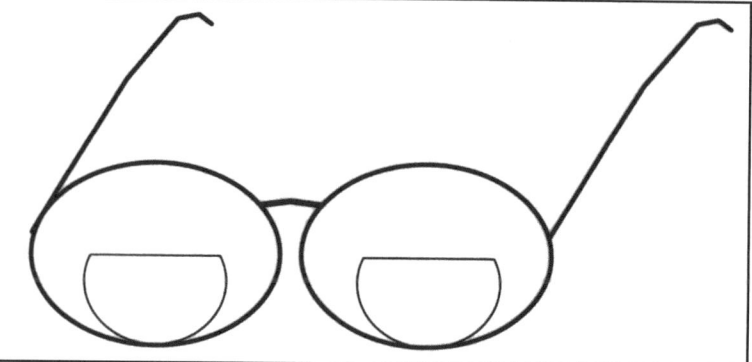

Figure 9-1. Most children's frames have a narrow enough eye size to enable the D-35 bifocal segment (which is 35 mm wide and shaped like a "D" on its side) to be used to treat high AC/A ratios without the child looking around the segment.

Children should be completely weaned from the bifocal by their early teen years. In order to accomplish this, the weaning process must start years before teen age, usually at around age 8 or 9. Incremental decreases in the add, while pushing plus in the distance as much as possible, should be made at every opportunity. Even new glasses that are lost going over the side of the boat should not be replaced exactly as they were; the add should be decreased slightly at every opportunity and at least yearly. When moderate hyperopia is corrected with contact lenses instead of spectacle correction, the need to accommodate at near is slightly decreased. Switching a young teen from glasses to contacts may eliminate the need for a low-power (+1.00) near add that had been necessary in the glasses.

Fresnel Press-Ons—Prisms and Spheres

More than 100 years ago, lighthouses were illuminated by a single candle with the help of the Fresnel principle—stacking prisms magnified the candle light so as to safely guide a ship or boat away from the rocky coast. The modern Fresnel press-on prism is a thin, inexpensive plastic piece that can be cut out and applied to existing glasses (or plano loaner glasses the patient has obtained from his or her favorite optical shop). Powers range from 1 prism diopter (PD) to 40 PD, although the higher numbers somewhat degrade visual acuity. Press-on prisms are a powerful tool in helping to determine a patient's fusional status once strabismus is "corrected" or in temporarily eliminating diplopia while a patient waits for recovery, change, or surgery. Certainly the most appreciative patients are those who come into the office with miserable diplopia and who leave fusing with single binocular vision restored. While press-on prisms may not be a permanent fix, they can eliminate costly errors in prescribing ground-in prism by allowing the patient to try the prism. They are invaluable for a patient whose condition is changing, such as a recovering cranial nerve palsy or Graves' restrictive ophthalmopathy. Fresnel press-ons are also a way to give two completely different prisms for the distance segment versus the near segment without compromising one for the other. Additionally, a single Fresnel prism can correct for both a horizontal and vertical deviation when applied at an angle.

Press-on spheres, although limited in power, allow a prescription to be changed temporarily, again avoiding the need for costly prescription changes. A decrease in power can be tried before weaning accommodative esotropes by adding minus press-ons. Plus lenses can be added for a patient who is cyclopleged for chronic iritis or to blur a dominant eye for amblyopia treatment in a patient with nystagmus. Traditional opaque occlusion often exacerbates nystagmus, but blurring the dominant eye with plus lenses (or graded Bangerter filters, which are explained later in this chapter) can be used to successfully treat amblyopia while minimizing the nystagmus.

Know Your Optical Shop

Get to know which optical shops, and specifically which opticians, are better at fitting children. The optical industry has changed over the years, becoming more of a business than a dispensary of visual aids. You will provide parents a real service if you can direct them to an optical shop with child-related warranties, a reasonable frame selection, and a child-friendly and patient optician. A good investment in children's eyewear will result in a child who is happy to wear the glasses, a parent who is happy to have his or her child wear the glasses, and an optical correction that makes the clinician happy.

The best warranty for children replaces a scratched lens and broken or damaged frame. A reasonable frame selection increases the chances of getting a good fit in a good-looking frame. Any optician will tell you that, up to a point, you get what you pay for. The better frames keep their adjustment longer and may hold up better. An optician who genuinely likes children will be more patient and answer parents' questions. Inevitably you will have questions for the optician when more difficult problems arise, such as when prescribing prisms, children's biofocals, or high-index lenses. It is also helpful for you to be familiar with your local charitable organizations that will help underwrite the cost of glasses for families in need.

Glasses for Children

Parents shudder at the thought of their beautiful baby in glasses. Of course, all children should be so lucky as to be able to have a problem that is fixable merely with glasses (as opposed to surgery) and to live in a society where the glasses are available to them. Instruct the parents regarding what to look for in a frame and in an optical shop. The size of the selection suggests the shop's experience with children. Ten children's frames versus 100 children's frames sends a clear message to the consumer: "We don't want to fit your child, so we carry only the barest minimum possible in hopes that one may fit," versus "We want your business and will probably be able to find a suitable frame for you." Some places welcome children and advertise it indirectly with their playroom (at their doctor's office), bag full of kid goodies (in grandma's pocketbook), or collection of kid-size tools and scraps (in uncle's workshop.) Parents have been avoiding child-unfriendly places since day one, whether it is a restaurant that is a little too quiet or an adult friend's house with lovely antiques and glassware on display. Remind parents that they may be visiting the optical shop a lot in the next few months and years, so it should be convenient to them with adequate parking and hours of operation.

Instruct the parent to look for a frame that sits comfortably on the child's face. The child should look more through the geometric center of the lens rather than the top edge of the frame, with most of the lens over his or her cheek (Figure 9-2). Spring hinges are now used on almost all children's frames. When a bifocal is prescribed to treat a high AC/A ratio (often associated with accommodative ET), show the parents with a drawing just where the line is intended to go, and explain why it is up much higher than an older presbyope's lens (Figure 9-3). Teaching the parents to be educated consumers is the best way to get appropriate glasses onto their children and increase the chances that their children will successfully wear the glasses.

Figure 9-2. This photo shows three children in good frame fits.

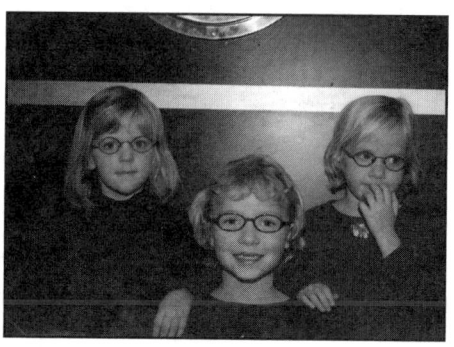

Figure 9-3. Instructions are helpful to both the optician and parent to show the proper bifocal segment height necessary to successfully treat a child with a high AC/A ratio.

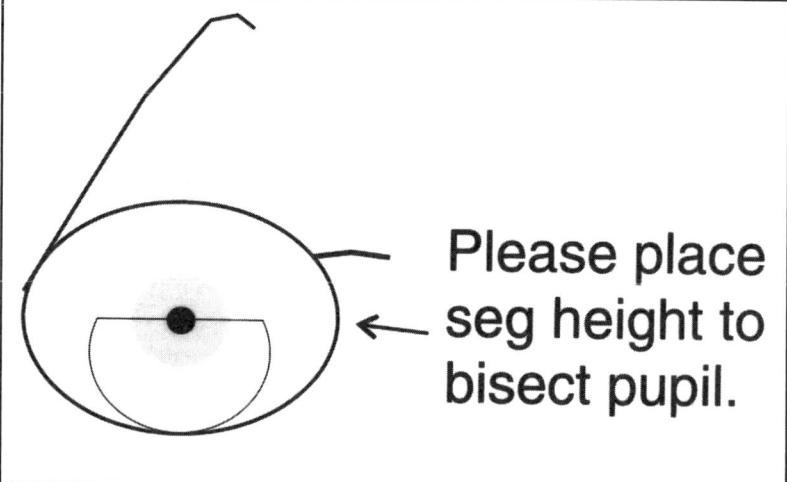

Amblyopia Treatment

Detection

Amblyopia treatment begins with early detection. Proper screening techniques must be understood by the pediatric and family practice office and by the early childhood screening systems within your state. Once the diagnosis is made, educating parents about the important role they play in making decisions for their child (who is too young to make a rational decision on his or her own behalf) is time well spent. Parents must understand that they are responsible for their child's treatment, which may include wearing glasses full-time as well as occlusion (which is frequently patching). The long-range scenario helps many parents grasp the importance of treating amblyopia in a young child. Patching is not forever and glasses may not be forever; blindness is.

Amblyopia Treatment Studies

The National Eye Institute has funded the Pediatric Eye Disease Investigator Group, known as PEDIG, to study different eye conditions and treatments affecting children. There have been several large multicenter investigations, including ones reviewing retinopathy of prematurity and the amblyopia treatment studies. Because of the ever-changing nature of evidence-based medicine, the best review of currently preferred practice managements may be found at http://public.pedig.jaeb.org.

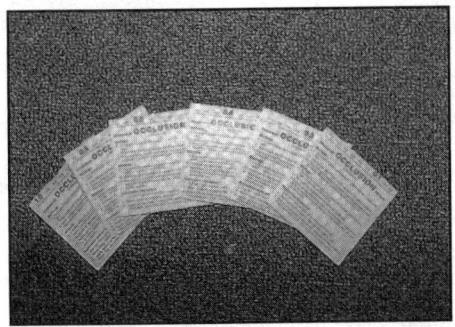

Figure 9-4. Bangerter filters are packaged in envelopes that are labeled by the amount of opacity.

Refractive Correction

Cycloplegic refractometry reveals both the refractive error of the two eyes and the difference between the two eyes. In the absence of strabismus, this difference must be balanced and adjusted. Prescribe the full amount of plus (push plus) for patients with esodeviations and consider reducing (cutting plus) for patients with exodeviations or ortho. The astigmatic error should be fully corrected and will be easily tolerated even by children who are first-time wearers.

Patching

The patch should be applied to the face (under the glasses) for the number of hours prescribed. No exceptions. When full-time occlusion is the initial treatment, careful follow-up appointments are critical to avoid the rare but disheartening occurrence of reverse or occlusion amblyopia. This happens when the good eye is patched too much, resulting in decreased vision in the initially better-seeing eye. A general rule of thumb in children who are patched full-time is to follow up in a certain number of weeks depending on their age in years—a 1-year-old child is rechecked in 1 week, a 2 year old in 2 weeks, etc—with no child ever going longer than 4 weeks. Follow-up visits may be stretched out when part-time occlusion is used. Parents must realize that a child is not having his or her amblyopia treated during sleep, even if the patch is on. In addition, clinicians should inquire about the number of hours a child actually spends swimming before casually saying that the child does not have to patch while swimming.

Filters

Bangerter filters, or foils, have revolutionized maintenance occlusion for children whose vision approaches normal and is nearly equal to the fellow eye (Figure 9-4). A filter is cut out and applied to the inside of the glasses lens over the dominant eye. The filters are graded according to the degree of opacity. A mildly opaque filter, a 0.8 for example, barely degrades the vision of the dominant eye, while a 0.4 filter will cut down the vision more significantly. When the child's vision is nearly equal, a 0.8 or 0.6 may be used; the denser 0.4 should be used if a difference of a few lines persists and is being treated. Because the child can easily look around the glasses lens (and the filter), foils are not usually useful in amblyopia worse than 10/40 or if a 0.4 foil must be resorted to in order to obtain initial results. Younger children may naturally look around the "dirty" lens. The foils are most useful in older children who have nearly equal vision, who understand the importance of treating their amblyopia, who have nearly straight eyes, and who are motivated to get rid of the patch. Since the filters are barely noticeable to anyone looking at the child, the success of this kind of occlusion therapy is not influenced by negative peer pressure, poor self-image, or teasing.

Pharmacological Penalization

Penalization by pharmacologically blurring the dominant eye only works if the dominant eye is significantly blurred by cycloplegia. If the dominant eye is plano or, worse, mildly myopic, cycloplegia will still allow that eye to have better vision than its amblyopic fellow. Even if the vision is worse in the cyclopleged dominant eye, many children with amblyopia will not switch over fixation to the amblyopic eye. Patients will tell you that 20/40 from an uncorrected refractive error is entirely different from 20/40 vision due to amblyopia. The side effects and implications of using drugs to treat a child who can be treated by other noninvasive methods must be considered by both the clinician and parents. Current recommendations may be found at PEDIG's Web site (http://public.pedig.jaeb.org).

Compliance

Stubborn children provide new challenges to the treatment of amblyopia. We all know them; I have a few who live right in my own home. These children will not brush their hair, will not let the peas touch the mashed potatoes, cannot stand the feel of ridges in their tube socks, and freak out when a 3-week-old bandage has to be removed from a wound that did not really exist in the first place. We clinicians smile sweetly and tell the exasperated parents that not only are full-time glasses in their immediate future but that their newly occluded child will not even be able to see (at first).

Parents have reacted to this news in a variety of ways ranging from crying, to laughing, to somberly just shaking their heads. It will be just one more battleground lodged somewhere in between the controversy over 1% versus 2% milk and finding the baseball cap that feels just right.

This is where the clinician and his or her support staff can do just that—provide support. Arming parents with helpful hints and your back line phone number will help. These parents understand the phrase "choose your battles," and in reality have made huge strides with their spirited children. Remind parents that their children do look twice before crossing the street, they do not play with light sockets, and they do keep their mittens on in sub-zero weather. The glasses and patch must be placed in the same category as these non-negotiable opportunities for confrontation. Ambiguous instructions are the very last thing these parents (and children) need to hear. "Do-it-and-get-it-over-with" works really well. It often helps the parents if the clinician tells the child the ground rules—no one touches the patch except the parents/caregivers who decide when the patch goes on and off. The patch is just like the medicine you would take for an ear infection. The doctor tells the parent what they need to use and how much of it and then the parent tells the child when it is time for medicine and ensures the child gets the appropriate amount. If it makes sense to the parent that he or she would never allow his or her child to go to the medication closet and help him- or herself to whatever medicine the child thought might work, then the parent will begin to see the ridiculousness of allowing a child to decide when he or she is through with the patch for the day. Express that it is the parents merely carrying out what the doctor, who went to school for a very long time to learn about these things, has decided will help the child.

Suggest that parents find a way to track success. Use a calendar with stickers for all the days the patching went well. A reward to look forward to helps even a small child get through the maze of stickers on his or her chart. Rewards can be simple—a trip to a favorite store, a new toy, a visit alone to Grandma's. Besides just complimenting them when they return, show the parents and child the results of their hard work. Saying that they have improved from 20/100 to 20/30 is not enough; show them the improvement using the eye chart. Of course the reward for doing well is usually that you get to do it more, but remind them that soon they will be able to switch to less patching or, using the drops less often, to a filter that will not show.

After treating hundreds of amblyopes, it is rare to find a child who just will not cooperate if the parents are determined and educated. Stubborn parents are a major cause of failure in treating amblyopic children. This is generally a result of the parents simply not understanding the importance of treating amblyopia and that it must be done before a certain age of visual maturity. That age, typically, is before a child can really make a rational decision to choose treatment for the improvement of his or her visual future. So the parents must make the choice. Graphically demonstrating poor vision to a person who has perfect vision may send the message home. Show the parent what the world looks like through +10 lenses. Another good technique is to show them arm restraints, both homemade and purchased (the more expensive, the better), that can be used so that the child cannot bend the elbow and remove the patch. Remind parents that a child with permanently poor vision in one eye will need safety eyewear at all times. Clinicians should certainly document when parents are noncompliant and some clinicians are actually insisting that parents sign-off on an eye in hopes of protecting themselves (the doctors) against future litigation by amblyopic adults who find themselves suddenly shut out of a career requiring good vision in each eye. This gets the point across to parents.

Esotropia Treatment

When glasses that correct hyperopia and high AC/A ratios alone do not work comfortably to straighten the eyes, fusion and/or divergence exercises may help to avoid surgery. While it is difficult to teach someone to diverge, it is possible to use base-in prism. Using a small, hand-held base-in prism while reading, however, will only work on patients with fusional capabilities, or fusion potential. Without fusion potential, surgery is the only alternative.

Divergence amplitudes are measured with base-in prism, and divergence is "taught" with base-in prism. It is often tempting to treat patients with esodeviations with base-out prism in their glasses correction. However, this in fact eliminates the patient's need to diverge altogether (even to get to the ortho position). Then, over time, the patient's divergence amplitudes invariably worsen, symptoms increase, and the patient needs more base-out prism in his or her glasses. The patient becomes completely dependent on the glasses and can never even consider contact lens correction. Many of these patients end up with a maximum amount of prism in their glasses, are still symptomatic, and ultimately require surgery.

Instead of giving constant base-out prism, give small amounts of base-in prism (to use strictly as an exercise), which will increase divergence amplitudes and ultimately increase their overall comfort. The prism can be increased in small increments as the patient is able to tolerate the new strain on the binocular visual system.

Other divergence exercises utilize the awareness of a near object outside of Panum's fusional space, such as bar reading or dot on the wall. Physiologic diplopia of a near object results when the patient views an object that is farther away. Maintaining focus on the distant object (the book being read or an imaginary place beyond the wall) while a near object (the pencil in front of the

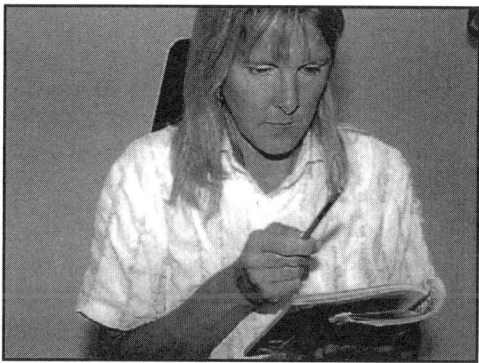 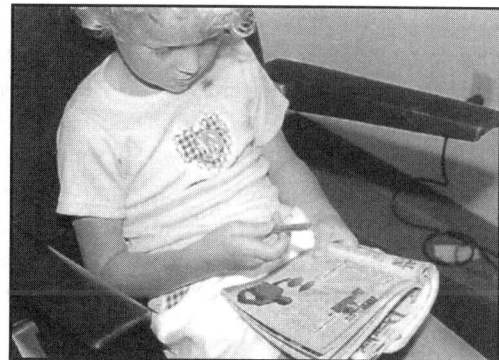

Figure 9-5. Bar reading is useful in improving divergence amplitudes and antisuppressing temporal retina. The head, the pencil, and the book are not moved. Only the eyes move across the line of text.

Figure 9-6. The dot-on-the-wall exercise utilizes physiological diplopia to build divergence amplitudes. The patient looks past the dot fixing at distance and sees two dots up close. As the patient backs away from the wall, fixation at far distance is more difficult to maintain as the two dots come closer together. The patient is instructed to get as far away from the wall as possible while still seeing two separate dots. Maximum distance would be 12 to 18 inches from the wall.

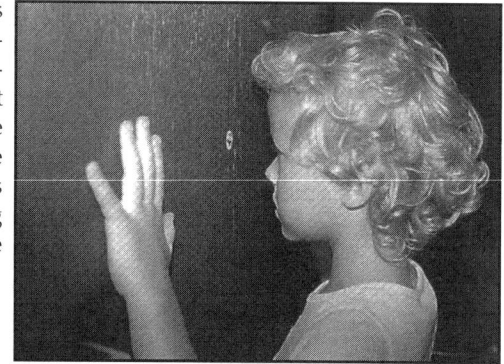

book or the dot on the wall) is perceived in crossed diplopia strengthens divergence, as the patient must avoid converging on the near object.

Bar reading is accomplished by reading a book with a pencil held vertically 5 or 6 inches in front of the page (Figure 9-5). Instruct the patient to not move the pencil, the page, or his or her head. The pencil should appear as two ghost images, neither of which will obliterate the print on the page if the patient is fusing (and diverging). If the patient begins suppressing one eye, one ghost image will disappear and the pencil will be seen singly by the other eye. This single image will block out part of the printed page.

The dot-on-the-wall exercise utilizes the same principle. A quarter-size dot is placed at eye level to the patient. The patient begins with his or her nose to the wall, fixating far off into the imaginary distance beyond the wall. The dot will appear in crossed diplopia. The patient should then slowly back away from the wall while maintaining distant focus and keeping the dot double (Figure 9-6). When the patient invariably converges on the dot, he or she should then press the nose against the wall and try again. Divergence is strengthened as the patient attempts to avoid converging on the dot. Success at the dot-on-the-wall exercise is measured in inches, and improvement in divergence amplitudes should result as the patient is able to get 12 or more inches away from the dot.

Red filters may be used to strengthen fusion because they provide an excellent obstacle to fusion. The patient is instructed to view a penlight and keep the light single as a red filter is introduced over one eye (Figure 9-7). As fusion with the red filter becomes easier in room light, the

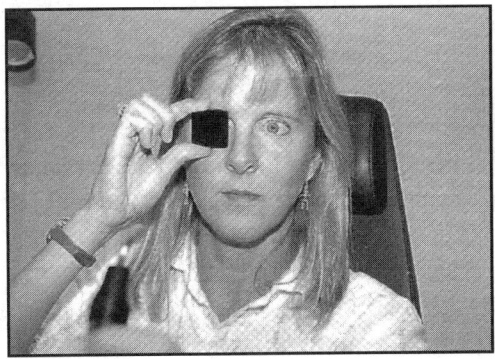

Figure 9-7. The red filter is placed over the dominant eye, and the patient looks at the fixation light. A patient with fusible strabismus who is tropic would see two lights, a red one and a white one. When a patient fuses, one pinkish light or red and white mixed together would be seen. If only one light is seen, either white or red, the deviating eye is being suppressed.

exercise is made more difficult by dimming the room lights. Performing the exercise in a darkened room makes it more difficult to fuse because there are no other clues to help keep the eyes straight. The goal is for the patient to maintain fusion even in a completely darkened room.

The Prism Adaptation Test (PAT) is sometimes used preoperatively to determine the amount of surgery that can be done on a patient with ET. Fully correcting base-out Fresnel press-on prisms are placed on a patient's glasses, or on loaner plano glasses, to be worn and rechecked hourly in the office or worn at home full time to be rechecked every few days. The deviation is remeasured through the Fresnel prism glasses. If an increase in the ET is found, it is counteracted with more base-out prism. The process is repeated until the patient no longer responds to the base-out prism by converging; instead of measuring ET through the base-out prism, the measurement is either ortho or exo. The final total amount of base-out prism is considered when surgical correction is planned.

Exodeviation Treatment

Again, everything depends on the patient's fusion potential. In the absence of fusion potential, only surgical intervention is likely to work. Of course, surgically straightening eyes that are accustomed to the exotropic position may result in diplopia for the patient with abnormal retinal correspondence (ARC).

When fusion does exist, a patient's symptoms (not necessarily the deviation) should be treated. When cosmesis is an added factor, a fusing patient who is aware of when the exotropia (XT) manifests itself—by appreciating diplopia—will know when to converge his or her eyes.

When poor convergence is the factor, convergence exercises usually work in the motivated patient. Reading or watching television with base-out prism improves convergence amplitudes while not allowing accommodative convergence to interfere with clarity. Simply doing "pencil push-ups" or NPC exercises does not separate the use of accommodative convergence from fusional convergence and, therefore, rarely works on the patient with true convergence insufficiency. The patient's visual requirements for convergence should be carefully assessed in addition to the measurement of his or her convergence. The convergence needs of an electrical engineer are different from those of a professional waterskier. Adequate convergence for one person may be too low and require treatment in another.

Young children may not be good candidates for active treatment of the exodeviation. The use of part-time occlusion may adequately improve their control until formal exercises can be initiated.[1]

Patients with exodeviations who can be taught to converge should not be given base-in prism in their glasses for comfort. Like the patients with esodeviations described earlier, the patients with exodeviations will also "eat up" the prism and completely lose their ability to converge at all, becoming completely dependent on their prism glasses and unable to wear contact lenses. While it may seem like the kind thing to do, giving base-in prism will backfire. The exception to this would be older patients who understand the situation and prefer expensive comfort over exercises. (Note: The cost of prismatic glasses that are created by only moving the optical centers should not cost more, as these glasses only require calculating the position of displacement.)

Many fusing patients with exodeviations actually are not bothered by the exodeviation. What disrupts fusion and drives the eye out is an accompanying vertical deviation. Treatment of the vertical deviation alone may eliminate the loss of fusion.

Hyperdeviation Treatment

Careful measurement and diagnosis of any vertical deviation are imperative. Treating a new hyper is not easily accomplished with exercises (red filter fusion or "stretching" the area of single binocular vision). However, a longstanding deviation that is starting to decompensate may actually respond to exercises. Vertical prism may eliminate the symptoms of decompensation, but the patient may come to depend on it. Many patients are unaware that holding their heads in a certain position will help them achieve binocularity. For example, a person with Graves' disease who cannot look up will be much happier driving the higher family minivan than the low-to-the-ground sports car. Sitting at the back of the theater, rather than down in the front, will also be more comfortable. The patient with a right superior oblique (RSO) palsy whose diplopia is worse to left gaze should sit on the left side of the theater/classroom/place of worship so as to force more looking into the remaining binocular field of right gaze. This may seem blatantly obvious to us, but to the elderly patient who has sat in the exact same pew for 45 years, a simple recommendation to move may significantly improve his or her life.

Diplopia Treatment

After determining the cause, treat the symptoms. Diplopia is always more bothersome when the images are together close enough to confuse the real object with the imposter. Diplopia may be treated with correcting prism, exercises when an area of fusion exists, head positioning to regain fusion, or occlusion. The occlusion may be as fancy as an opaque iris painted on a contact lens or as simple as closing one eye when necessary. Determine the real complaints and problems of the patient and work to solve them, not the ones on your own agenda. While I would personally like to see every patient have binocularity and fusion, that is not a best option for every patient. Some patients may be able to successfully occlude themselves by closing one eye intermittently to determine the real object. Others may need full-time occlusion. Some patients will care about cosmesis, some will not. Dense Bangerter filters may adequately hide the extra image while preserving good cosmesis for the patient. Appropriate treatment results in tolerable symptoms for the patient.

Reference

1. Freeman RS, Isenberg SJ. The use of part-time occlusion for early onset unilateral exotropia. *J Pediatr Ophthalmol Strabismus*. 1989;26(2):94-95.

Appendix

High refractive errors change the actual amount of deviation from the amount traditionally measured with prisms. Tables A-1 and A-2 show the adjustments needed to accurately provide measurements on patients with strabismus and high myopia or hyperopia.

Table A-1
Myopic Spectacle Power (D)

Measured Tropia (△)	-1	-2	-3	-4	-5	-6	-7	-8	-9	-10	-12	-15	-20	-30
5	5	5	5	5	4	4	4	4	4	4	4	4	3	3
10	10	10	9	9	9	9	9	8	8	8	8	7	7	6
15	15	14	14	14	13	13	13	12	12	12	12	11	10	9
20	20	19	19	18	18	17	17	17	16	16	15	15	13	11
25	24	24	23	23	22	22	21	21	20	20	19	18	17	14
30	29	29	28	27	27	26	26	25	24	24	23	22	20	17
35	34	33	33	32	31	30	30	30	29	28	27	25	23	20
40	39	38	37	36	36	35	34	33	33	32	31	29	26	23
45	44	43	42	41	40	39	38	37	37	36	35	33	30	26
50	49	48	47	45	44	43	43	42	41	40	38	36	33	29
60	59	57	56	55	53	52	51	50	49	48	46	44	40	34
70	68	67	65	64	62	61	60	58	57	56	54	51	46	40

This table calculates the true deviation measured in a myopic patient wearing spectacles. Find the spectacle power across the top and the deviation measured along the side, and the resultant tropia in the intersecting box is the true deviation, ET, XT, or HT. (Reprinted with permission from Hansen VC. Common pitfalls in measuring strabismic patients. Am Orthoptic J. 1989;39:3-11.)

Table A-2
Hyperopic Spectacle Power (D)

Measured Tropia (△)	+1	+2	+3	+4	+5	+6	+7	+8	+9	+10	+12	+15	+20	+30
5	5	5	5	6	6	6	6	6	6	7	7	8	10	20
10	10	11	11	11	11	12	12	13	13	13	14	16	20	40
15	15	16	16	16	17	18	18	19	19	20	21	24	30	60
20	21	21	22	22	23	24	24	25	26	27	29	32	40	80
25	26	26	27	28	29	29	30	31	32	33	36	40	50	100
30	31	32	32	33	34	35	36	38	39	40	43	48	60	120
35	36	37	38	39	40	41	42	44	45	47	50	56	70	140
40	41	42	43	44	46	47	48	50	52	53	57	64	80	160
45	46	47	49	50	51	53	55	56	58	60	64	72	90	180
50	51	53	54	56	57	59	61	63	65	67	71	80	100	200
60	62	63	65	67	69	71	73	75	77	80	87	96	120	240
70	72	74	76	78	80	82	85	88	90	93	100	112	140	280

This table calculates the true deviation measured in a hypermetropic patient wearing spectacles. Find the spectacle power across the top and the deviation measured along the side, and the resultant tropia in the intersecting box is the true deviation, ET, XT, or HT. (Reprinted with permission from Hansen VC. Common pitfalls in measuring strabismic patients. Am Orthoptic J. 1989;39:3-11.)

Index

WAIT
...There's More!

Certified Ophthalmic Assistant Exam Review Manual, Second Edition
Janice K. Ledford, COMT
192 pp., Soft Cover, 2003,
ISBN 13: 978-1-55642-642-1, Order# 66429, **$44.95**

This is an essential resource for anyone preparing to become certified as an ophthalmic assistant. With over 650 exam-style questions and explanatory answers, illustrations, and photographs, this user-friendly text is excellent for both learning and reviewing important eyecare topics. Subjects include taking a patient history, lensometry, measuring intraocular pressure, understanding optics, and much more.

Certified Ophthalmic Technician Exam Review Manual, Second Edition
Janice K. Ledford, COMT
272 pp., Soft Cover, 2004,
ISBN 13: 978-1-55642-648-3, Order# 66488, **$44.95**

This text delivers the essentials you need for certification as an ophthalmic technician. Updated to include the latest JCAHPO® criteria, this helpful resource contains over 1,300 exam-style questions and explanatory answers covering everything you need to know. This is an excellent learning text for students seeking to develop their knowledge in the field of eyecare as well as a useful reference for physicians.

The Little Eye Book: A Pupil's Guide to Understanding Ophthalmology, Second Edition
Janice K. Ledford, COMT
192 pp., Soft Cover, 2009,
ISBN 13: 978-1-55642-884-5, Order# 68845, **$23.95**

This text is an easy-to-understand introduction to the field of eyecare that has been updated into a new *Second Edition*. This book is written with the non-physician in mind, so you won't be bogged down with heavy details, yet every basic fact that you need is right here. With photographs as well as drawings, helpful tables, and charts, this conversational-style text packs a big punch.

Quick Reference Dictionary of Eyecare Terminology, Fifth Edition
Janice K. Ledford, COMT; Joseph Hoffman
504 pp., Soft Cover, 2008,
ISBN 13: 978-1-55642-805-0, Order# 68057, **$35.95**

A leading resource for nearly two decades and a daily reference for thousands of eyecare professionals, this text continues the tradition and provides the latest terms, concepts, conditions, and important resources in an instant. Compact, concise, and informative, this *Fifth Edition* provides quick access to over 3,700 terms and their definitions, including over 400 new words.

Please visit
www.slackbooks.com
to order any of these titles!
24 Hours a Day...7 Days a Week!

Attention Industry Partners!

Whether you are interested in buying multiple copies of a book, chapter reprints, or looking for something new and different—we are able to accommodate your needs.

Multiple Copies

At attractive discounts starting for purchases as low as 25 copies for a single title, SLACK Incorporated will be able to meet all of your needs.

Chapter Reprints

SLACK Incorporated is able to offer the chapters you want in a format that will lead to success. Bound with an attractive cover, use the chapters that are a fit specifically for your company. Available for quantities of 100 or more.

Customize

SLACK Incorporated is able to create a specialized custom version of any of our products specifically for your company.

Please contact the Marketing Communications Director of Health Care Books and Journals for further details on multiple copy purchases, chapter reprints or custom printing at 1-800-257-8290 or 1-856-848-1000.

Please note all conditions are subject to change.

CODE: 328

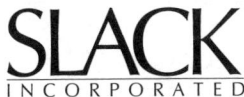

SLACK Incorporated • Health Care Books and Journals
6900 Grove Road • Thorofare, NJ 08086

1-800-257-8290 or 1-856-848-1000

Fax: 1-856-848-6091 • E-mail: orders@slackinc.com • Visit: www.slackbooks.com